Welcome to the **_"DASH Diet Cookbook for Renal Health: Maintaining Renal Health with Easy and Delicious DASH Diet Meals."_** This book is your comprehensive guide to a healthier lifestyle, designed specifically to support kidney health through the renowned DASH (Dietary Approaches to Stop Hypertension) diet. Whether you are managing a renal condition or simply aiming to maintain optimal kidney function, the recipes and information contained within these pages will empower you to make nutritious and delicious choices every day.

Understanding the Importance of Renal Health

Your kidneys play a crucial role in maintaining overall health by filtering waste products and excess fluids from your blood, regulating blood pressure, balancing electrolytes, and supporting red blood cell production. However, kidney disease and other renal conditions can compromise these essential functions, leading to serious health complications. Diet is a powerful tool in managing and preventing kidney disease, and the DASH diet has been recognized for its benefits in promoting cardiovascular and renal health.

What is the DASH Diet?

The DASH diet emphasizes the consumption of whole foods rich in nutrients like potassium, calcium, and magnesium while reducing sodium intake. This balanced approach not only helps manage blood pressure but also supports kidney health by reducing the strain on these vital organs. The DASH diet includes a variety of fruits, vegetables, whole grains, lean proteins, and low-fat dairy, making it a versatile and enjoyable way to eat healthily.

Why This Cookbook?

This cookbook is specially crafted to meet the unique dietary needs of those focused on renal health. With over 110 easy and delicious recipes, you will find meals that are not only kidney-friendly but also satisfying and flavorful. Each recipe is carefully developed to align with the principles of the DASH diet, ensuring that you get the right nutrients without compromising on taste.

What to Expect

In this book, you will discover a wide range of recipes, from hearty breakfasts and wholesome lunches to delightful dinners and indulgent desserts. We have also included helpful tips on meal planning, grocery shopping, and cooking techniques to make your culinary journey enjoyable and stress-free. Whether you are new to the DASH diet or looking to expand your recipe repertoire, this cookbook will be your trusted companion in the kitchen.

1. Oatmeal with Fresh Berries

Ingredient:

- 1 cup old•fashioned oats
- 1 1/2 cups unsweetened almond milk or low•fat milk
- 1/2 cup fresh blueberries
- 1/2 cup fresh raspberries
- 1 tbsp honey (optional)
- Cinnamon to taste

Instructions:
1. In a medium saucepan, bring the milk to a simmer over medium heat.

2. Add the oats and cook, stirring occasionally, for 5•7 minutes until the oats are tender and the mixture has thickened.

3. Remove from heat and stir in the fresh berries.

4. If desired, drizzle with a small amount of honey and sprinkle with cinnamon.

This recipe is DASH diet•friendly because:
- It uses whole grain oats, which are high in fiber and low in sodium.

- It incorporates fresh, low•sodium berries as the primary sweetener.

- It uses low•fat or unsweetened almond milk, which is low in sodium and saturated fat.

- The optional honey provides a small amount of sweetness without excessive added sugar.

This recipe is also suitable for renal health because:
- It is low in sodium, which is important for managing blood pressure and kidney function.

- The berries are low in potassium, making this a good choice for those with kidney disease.

- The oats and milk provide protein and complex carbohydrates without excessive amounts of phosphorus.

Enjoy this nutritious and delicious breakfast option!

2. Greek Yogurt with Honey and Nuts

Ingredient:

• 1 cup plain, unsweetened Greek yogurt
• 1 tbsp raw, unprocessed honey
• 2 tbsp chopped walnuts or almonds

Instructions:

1. Spoon the Greek yogurt into a serving bowl.

2. Drizzle the honey over the top of the yogurt.

3. Sprinkle the chopped nuts over the honey.

This recipe is DASH diet•friendly because:

• It uses plain, unsweetened Greek yogurt, which is high in protein and low in sodium.

• The honey provides a natural sweetener without excessive added sugar.

• The nuts add healthy fats and fiber without too much sodium.

This recipe is also suitable for renal health because:

• The Greek yogurt is a good source of protein without excessive amounts of phosphorus.

• The honey and nuts are low in potassium, making this a good choice for those with kidney disease.

• The overall sodium content is low, which is important for managing blood pressure and kidney function.

Enjoy this simple, nutritious, and delicious snack or light meal!

3. Whole Grain Toast with Avocado

Ingredient:

- 2 slices of whole grain or sprouted bread
- 1/2 ripe avocado, mashed
- 1 tbsp fresh lemon juice
- 1/4 tsp ground black pepper
- Pinch of salt (optional)

Instructions:

1. Toast the whole grain or sprouted bread until lightly golden.

2. In a small bowl, mash the avocado with the lemon juice, black pepper, and a pinch of salt (if using).

3. Spread the mashed avocado evenly over the toasted bread slices.

This recipe is DASH diet•friendly because:

- It uses whole grain or sprouted bread, which is high in fiber and low in sodium.

- The avocado provides healthy monounsaturated fats without excessive sodium.

- The lemon juice and black pepper add flavor without the need for added salt.

This recipe is also suitable for renal health because:

- The whole grain bread and avocado are low in potassium, making this a good choice for those with kidney disease.

- The overall sodium content is low, which is important for managing blood pressure and kidney function.

- The healthy fats and fiber from the avocado and whole grains can help support overall health.

Enjoy this simple, nutritious, and delicious snack or light meal!

4. Egg White Omelet with Spinach and Tomatoes

Ingredient:

• 4 egg whites
• 1 cup fresh spinach, chopped
• 1/2 cup cherry tomatoes, halved
• 1 tbsp low•fat or non•fat milk
• 1/4 tsp ground black pepper
• Pinch of salt (optional)

Instructions:
1. In a small bowl, whisk together the egg whites and milk until well combined.

2. Spray a non•stick skillet with cooking spray and heat over medium heat.

3. Pour the egg white mixture into the skillet and let it cook for 2•3 minutes, or until the bottom is set.

4. Sprinkle the chopped spinach and halved cherry tomatoes over the top of the egg whites.

5. Fold the omelet in half and continue cooking for another 2•3 minutes, or until the egg whites are fully cooked.

6. Slide the omelet onto a plate and season with black pepper and a pinch of salt (if using).

This recipe is DASH diet•friendly because:
• It uses egg whites, which are low in sodium and high in protein.

• The spinach and tomatoes provide a variety of vitamins, minerals, and antioxidants without excessive sodium. The small amount of milk adds a creamy texture without too much saturated fat.

This recipe is also suitable for renal health because:
• The egg whites, spinach, and tomatoes are all low in potassium, making this a good choice for those with kidney disease.

• The overall sodium content is low, which is important for managing blood pressure and kidney function. The protein from the egg whites can help support muscle health and overall nutrition.

5. Smoothie with Almond Milk, Spinach, and Banana

Ingredient:

- 1 cup unsweetened almond milk
- 1 cup fresh spinach, packed
- 1 ripe banana, frozen
- 1 tbsp ground flaxseed (optional)
- 1 tsp honey (optional)

Instructions:

1. In a high•speed blender, combine the almond milk, spinach, frozen banana, and ground flaxseed (if using).

2. Blend on high speed until the mixture is smooth and creamy, about 1•2 minutes.

3. If desired, add a teaspoon of honey and blend again briefly to incorporate.

This recipe is DASH diet•friendly because:

• It uses unsweetened almond milk, which is low in sodium and saturated fat.

• The spinach and banana provide natural sweetness and a variety of vitamins and minerals without added sugars.

• The optional ground flaxseed adds healthy omega•3 fatty acids and fiber.

This recipe is also suitable for renal health because:

• The almond milk, spinach, and banana are all relatively low in potassium, making this a good choice for those with kidney disease.

• The overall sodium content is low, which is important for managing blood pressure and kidney function.

• The protein, fiber, and healthy fats in this smoothie can help support overall nutrition and health.

Enjoy this refreshing and nutritious smoothie as a snack or light meal!

6. Low•Fat Cottage Cheese with Pineapple

Ingredient:

• 1 cup low•fat or non•fat cottage cheese
• 1/2 cup fresh pineapple, diced
• 1 tsp honey (optional)
• Ground cinnamon (optional)

Instructions:
1. In a small bowl, combine the low•fat or non•fat cottage cheese and diced pineapple.

2. If desired, drizzle the honey over the top and sprinkle with a dash of ground cinnamon.

This recipe is DASH diet•friendly because:

• It uses low•fat or non•fat cottage cheese, which is high in protein and low in sodium and saturated fat.

• The fresh pineapple provides natural sweetness without added sugars.

• The optional honey provides a small amount of sweetness without excessive added sugar.

This recipe is also suitable for renal health because:

• The cottage cheese and pineapple are both relatively low in potassium, making this a good choice for those with kidney disease.

• The overall sodium content is low, which is important for managing blood pressure and kidney function.

• The protein from the cottage cheese can help support muscle health and overall nutrition.

Enjoy this simple, nutritious, and delicious snack or light meal!

7. Quinoa Breakfast Bowl with Blueberries

Ingredient:

• 1/2 cup cooked quinoa, cooled
• 1/2 cup unsweetened almond milk
• 1/2 cup fresh blueberries
• 1 tbsp chopped walnuts or almonds
• 1 tsp honey (optional)
• Ground cinnamon (optional)

Instructions:

1. In a medium bowl, combine the cooked quinoa and unsweetened almond milk.

2. Top the quinoa mixture with the fresh blueberries and chopped nuts.

3. If desired, drizzle the honey over the top and sprinkle with a dash of ground cinnamon.

This recipe is DASH diet•friendly because:

• It uses quinoa, which is a whole grain that is high in fiber and protein.

• The unsweetened almond milk is low in sodium and saturated fat.

• The blueberries provide natural sweetness and antioxidants without added sugars.

• The optional honey provides a small amount of sweetness without excessive added sugar.

This recipe is also suitable for renal health because:

• The quinoa, blueberries, and almond milk are all relatively low in potassium, making this a good choice for those with kidney disease.

• The overall sodium content is low, which is important for managing blood pressure and kidney function.

• The protein, fiber, and healthy fats in this breakfast bowl can help support overall nutrition and health.

Enjoy this nutritious and delicious start to your day!

8. Whole Wheat English Muffin with Almond Butter

Ingredient:

• 1 whole wheat English muffin
• 2 tbsp natural, unsalted almond butter
• 1 tsp honey (optional)

Instructions:
1. Toast the whole wheat English muffin until lightly golden.

2. Spread the almond butter evenly over the muffin halves.

3. If desired, drizzle a small amount of honey over the almond butter.

This recipe is DASH diet·friendly because:

• It uses a whole wheat English muffin, which is a whole grain that is high in fiber and low in sodium.

• The natural, unsalted almond butter provides healthy fats and protein without excessive sodium.

• The optional honey provides a small amount of sweetness without added sugars.

This recipe is also suitable for renal health because:

• The whole wheat English muffin and almond butter are both relatively low in potassium, making this a good choice for those with kidney disease.

• The overall sodium content is low, which is important for managing blood pressure and kidney function.

• The protein, fiber, and healthy fats in this snack can help support overall nutrition and health.

Enjoy this simple, nutritious, and delicious snack or light meal!

9. Apple Slices with Peanut Butter

Ingredient:

• 1 medium apple, sliced
• 2 tbsp natural, unsalted peanut butter

Instructions:
1. Wash and slice the apple into thin wedges.

2. Spread the peanut butter evenly over the apple slices.

This recipe is DASH diet•friendly because:

• It uses a fresh, whole fruit (apple) as the base, which is high in fiber and low in sodium.

• The natural, unsalted peanut butter provides healthy fats and protein without excessive sodium.

This recipe is also suitable for renal health because:

• Apples are relatively low in potassium, making this a good choice for those with kidney disease.

• The peanut butter is also low in potassium, and the overall sodium content is low, which is important for managing blood pressure and kidney function.

• The combination of fiber, protein, and healthy fats can help support overall nutrition and health.

Enjoy this simple, nutritious, and delicious snack!

10. Low-Sodium Turkey Bacon with Scrambled Egg Whites

Ingredient:

• 2 slices low•sodium turkey bacon
• 2 egg whites
• 1 tbsp low•fat or non•fat milk
• Ground black pepper to taste

Instructions:
1. In a non•stick skillet, cook the low•sodium turkey bacon over medium heat until crispy, about 3•4 minutes per side. Transfer to a paper towel•lined plate.

2. In a small bowl, whisk together the egg whites and milk.

3. Spray the same skillet with cooking spray and heat over medium heat.

4. Pour the egg white mixture into the skillet and cook, stirring occasionally, until the eggs are fully cooked and scrambled, about 2•3 minutes.

5. Serve the scrambled egg whites alongside the low•sodium turkey bacon. Season with ground black pepper to taste.

This recipe is DASH diet•friendly because:

• It uses low•sodium turkey bacon, which is lower in sodium than traditional pork bacon.

• The egg whites are a lean protein source that is low in sodium and saturated fat.

• The small amount of milk adds creaminess without excessive sodium or saturated fat.

This recipe is also suitable for renal health because:

• The low•sodium turkey bacon and egg whites are both relatively low in potassium, making this a good choice for those with kidney disease.

• The overall sodium content is low, which is important for managing blood pressure and kidney function.

• The protein from the egg whites can help support muscle health and overall nutrition.

11. Carrot Sticks with Hummus

Ingredient:

• 1 cup baby carrots or carrot sticks
• 2 tbsp traditional or roasted red pepper hummus

Instructions:

1. Wash and peel the carrots, if desired, and cut into sticks or leave whole as baby carrots.

2. Serve the carrot sticks alongside the hummus for dipping.

This recipe is DASH diet•friendly because:

• Carrots are a low•sodium, high•fiber vegetable that is rich in vitamins and minerals.

• Hummus is a plant•based dip that is high in protein, fiber, and healthy fats without excessive sodium.

This recipe is also suitable for renal health because:

• Carrots are relatively low in potassium, making them a good choice for those with kidney disease.

• The hummus is also low in potassium, and the overall sodium content is low, which is important for managing blood pressure and kidney function.

• The combination of fiber, protein, and healthy fats can help support overall nutrition and health.

Enjoy this simple, nutritious, and delicious snack!

12. Celery with Low•Sodium Peanut Butter

Ingredient:

• 2•3 celery stalks, cut into 3•4 inch pieces
• 2 tbsp low•sodium peanut butter

Instructions:

1. Wash and cut the celery stalks into 3•4 inch pieces.

2. Spread the low•sodium peanut butter evenly over the celery sticks.

This recipe is DASH diet•friendly because:

• Celery is a low•sodium, high•fiber vegetable that is rich in vitamins and minerals.

• The low•sodium peanut butter provides healthy fats and protein without excessive sodium.

This recipe is also suitable for renal health because:

• Celery is relatively low in potassium, making it a good choice for those with kidney disease.

• The low•sodium peanut butter is also low in potassium, and the overall sodium content is low, which is important for managing blood pressure and kidney function.

• The combination of fiber, protein, and healthy fats can help support overall nutrition and health.

Enjoy this simple, nutritious, and delicious snack!

13. Sliced Cucumbers with Greek Yogurt Dip

Ingredient:

- 1 medium cucumber, sliced
- 1/2 cup plain, unsweetened Greek yogurt
- 1 tbsp fresh dill, chopped (or 1 tsp dried dill)
- 1 tbsp lemon juice
- 1/4 tsp garlic powder
- Ground black pepper to taste

Instructions:

1. Wash and slice the cucumber into thin rounds or half•moons.

2. In a small bowl, mix together the Greek yogurt, fresh dill (or dried dill), lemon juice, and garlic powder. Season with ground black pepper to taste.

3. Serve the cucumber slices alongside the Greek yogurt dip for dipping.

This recipe is DASH diet•friendly because:

- Cucumbers are a low•sodium, high•fiber vegetable that is rich in vitamins and minerals.

- The plain, unsweetened Greek yogurt is a high•protein, low•sodium dairy product.

- The dill, lemon juice, and garlic powder add flavor without the need for excessive sodium.

This recipe is also suitable for renal health because:

- Cucumbers and Greek yogurt are both relatively low in potassium, making this a good choice for those with kidney disease.

- The overall sodium content is low, which is important for managing blood pressure and kidney function.

- The protein and healthy fats in the Greek yogurt can help support overall nutrition and health.

Enjoy this refreshing and nutritious snack!

14. Fresh Fruit Salad

Ingredient:

- 1 cup diced pineapple
- 1 cup diced strawberries
- 1 cup diced cantaloupe or honeydew melon
- 1/2 cup blueberries
- 1 tbsp fresh lemon juice
- 1 tsp honey (optional)

Instructions:

1. In a large bowl, combine the diced pineapple, strawberries, cantaloupe/honeydew, and blueberries.

2. Drizzle the lemon juice over the fruit and gently toss to coat.

3. If desired, drizzle the honey over the fruit salad and toss lightly to combine.

This recipe is DASH diet•friendly because:

- It uses a variety of fresh, whole fruits that are low in sodium and high in fiber, vitamins, and minerals.

- The lemon juice provides a natural source of acidity without the need for added sugars or sodium.

- The optional honey provides a small amount of sweetness without excessive added sugar.

This recipe is also suitable for renal health because:

- The fruits used in this salad are relatively low in potassium, making it a good choice for those with kidney disease.

- The overall sodium content is low, which is important for managing blood pressure and kidney function.

- The natural sugars, fiber, and vitamins in the fruit can help support overall nutrition and health.

15. Air•Popped Popcorn with Olive Oil

Ingredient:

• 1/4 cup unpopped popcorn kernels
• 1 tsp extra•virgin olive oil
• Ground black pepper (optional)

Instructions:

1. In an air popper, pop the unpopped popcorn kernels according to the manufacturer's instructions.

2. Once the popcorn is popped, transfer it to a large bowl.

3. Drizzle the extra•virgin olive oil over the popcorn and toss to coat evenly.

4. If desired, season the popcorn with a light sprinkle of ground black pepper.

This recipe is DASH diet•friendly because:

• Air•popped popcorn is a whole grain that is low in sodium and high in fiber.

• The extra•virgin olive oil provides healthy monounsaturated fats without excessive sodium.

• The optional black pepper adds flavor without the need for added salt.

This recipe is also suitable for renal health because:

• Popcorn is relatively low in potassium, making it a good choice for those with kidney disease.

• The olive oil is also low in potassium, and the overall sodium content is low, which is important for managing blood pressure and kidney function.

• The fiber and healthy fats in this snack can help support overall nutrition and health.

Enjoy this simple, nutritious, and delicious snack!

16. Handful of Unsalted Nuts

Ingredient:

• 1/4 cup mixed unsalted nuts (such as almonds, walnuts, cashews, or pistachios)

Instructions:
1. Measure out a 1/4 cup portion of your desired unsalted nuts.

2. Enjoy the nuts as a snack.

This recipe is DASH diet•friendly because:

• Unsalted nuts are a source of healthy fats, protein, and fiber without excessive sodium.

• The variety of nuts provides a range of beneficial nutrients.

This recipe is also suitable for renal health because:

• Nuts are relatively low in potassium, making them a good choice for those with kidney disease.

• The lack of added salt means the overall sodium content is low, which is important for managing blood pressure and kidney function.

• The healthy fats, protein, and fiber in nuts can help support overall nutrition and health.

Enjoy this simple, nutritious, and satisfying snack!

17. Bell Pepper Strips with Guacamole

Ingredient:

- 1 medium bell pepper, sliced into strips
- 1 ripe avocado, mashed
- 1 tbsp fresh lime juice
- 2 tbsp diced onion
- 1 tbsp chopped cilantro (optional)
- 1/4 tsp ground cumin
- Salt and pepper to taste

Instructions:

1. Wash and slice the bell pepper into long, thin strips.

2. In a small bowl, mash the avocado with the lime juice, onion, cilantro (if using), and cumin. Season with a pinch of salt and pepper to taste.

3. Serve the bell pepper strips alongside the guacamole for dipping.

This recipe is DASH diet•friendly because:

- Bell peppers are a low•sodium, high•fiber vegetable that is rich in vitamins and minerals.

- Avocado provides healthy monounsaturated fats without excessive sodium.

- The lime juice, onion, and cilantro add flavor without the need for added salt.

This recipe is also suitable for renal health because:

- Bell peppers and avocado are both relatively low in potassium, making this a good choice for those with kidney disease.

- The overall sodium content is low, which is important for managing blood pressure and kidney function.

- The healthy fats, fiber, and nutrients in this snack can help support overall nutrition and health.

Enjoy this refreshing and nutritious snack!

18. Low•Fat Cheese with Whole Grain Crackers

Ingredient:

• 1 oz low•fat cheddar or Swiss cheese, sliced or cubed
• 6•8 whole grain crackers

Instructions:
1. Arrange the low•fat cheese slices or cubes on a plate.

2. Serve the cheese alongside the whole grain crackers.

This recipe is DASH diet•friendly because:

• Low•fat cheese is a good source of protein and calcium without excessive saturated fat or sodium.

• Whole grain crackers are a high•fiber, low•sodium carbohydrate source.

This recipe is also suitable for renal health because:

• Low•fat cheese and whole grain crackers are both relatively low in potassium, making this a good choice for those with kidney disease.

• The overall sodium content is low, which is important for managing blood pressure and kidney function.

• The combination of protein, fiber, and complex carbohydrates can help support overall nutrition and health.

Enjoy this simple, nutritious, and satisfying snack!

19. Cherry Tomatoes with Balsamic Drizzle

Ingredient:

- 1 cup cherry tomatoes, halved
- 1 tbsp balsamic vinegar
- 1 tsp extra•virgin olive oil
- 1 tsp fresh basil, chopped (optional)
- Ground black pepper to taste

Instructions:

1. In a small bowl, combine the halved cherry tomatoes, balsamic vinegar, and olive oil. Toss gently to coat the tomatoes.

2. If desired, sprinkle the chopped fresh basil over the tomatoes.

3. Season with ground black pepper to taste.

This recipe is DASH diet•friendly because:

- Cherry tomatoes are a low•sodium, high•fiber vegetable that is rich in vitamins and antioxidants.

- Balsamic vinegar and olive oil provide flavor without the need for added salt.

- The optional fresh basil adds additional flavor without increasing the sodium content.

This recipe is also suitable for renal health because:

- Cherry tomatoes are relatively low in potassium, making them a good choice for those with kidney disease.

- The overall sodium content is low, which is important for managing blood pressure and kidney function.

- The natural sugars, fiber, and nutrients in the tomatoes can help support overall nutrition and health.

Enjoy this simple, refreshing, and nutritious snack or side dish!

20. Edamame

Ingredient:

• 1 cup frozen, shelled edamame
• 1 tsp low•sodium soy sauce (optional)
• Ground black pepper to taste

Instructions:

1. Bring a medium pot of water to a boil.

2. Add the frozen, shelled edamame and cook for 3•5 minutes, until tender.

3. Drain the edamame and transfer to a serving bowl.

4. If desired, drizzle the low•sodium soy sauce over the edamame and toss to coat.

5. Season with ground black pepper to taste.

This recipe is DASH diet•friendly because:

• Edamame is a low•sodium, high•fiber, and high•protein legume that is rich in vitamins and minerals.

• The optional low•sodium soy sauce provides flavor without excessive sodium.

• The black pepper adds flavor without the need for added salt.

This recipe is also suitable for renal health because:

• Edamame is relatively low in potassium, making it a good choice for those with kidney disease.

• The overall sodium content is low, which is important for managing blood pressure and kidney function.

• The protein, fiber, and nutrients in edamame can help support overall nutrition and health.

Enjoy this simple, nutritious, and delicious snack!

21. Spinach Salad with Strawberries and Walnuts

Ingredient:

• 2 cups fresh spinach, washed and dried
• 1/2 cup fresh strawberries, sliced
• 2 tbsp chopped walnuts
• 1 tbsp balsamic vinegar
• 1 tsp extra•virgin olive oil
• Ground black pepper to taste

Instructions:
1. In a large salad bowl, combine the fresh spinach, sliced strawberries, and chopped walnuts.

2. In a small bowl, whisk together the balsamic vinegar and olive oil.

3. Drizzle the vinaigrette over the salad and toss gently to coat.

4. Season with ground black pepper to taste.

This recipe is DASH diet•friendly because:

• Spinach is a low•sodium, high•fiber, and nutrient•dense green.

• Strawberries provide natural sweetness and antioxidants without added sugars.

• Walnuts are a source of healthy fats and protein without excessive sodium.

• The balsamic vinegar and olive oil dressing adds flavor without the need for added salt.

This recipe is also suitable for renal health because:

• Spinach, strawberries, and walnuts are all relatively low in potassium, making this a good choice for those with kidney disease.

• The overall sodium content is low, which is important for managing blood pressure and kidney function.

• The combination of fiber, healthy fats, and nutrients can help support overall nutrition and health.

22. Greek Salad with Cucumber, Tomato, and Feta

Ingredient:

• 1 cup diced cucumber
• 1 cup diced tomatoes
• 2 tbsp crumbled low•fat feta cheese
• 1 tbsp red wine vinegar
• 1 tsp extra•virgin olive oil
• 1 tsp dried oregano
• Ground black pepper to taste

Instructions:

1. In a medium bowl, combine the diced cucumber, diced tomatoes, and crumbled low•fat feta cheese.

2. In a small bowl, whisk together the red wine vinegar and olive oil.

3. Drizzle the vinaigrette over the salad and toss gently to coat.

4. Sprinkle the dried oregano over the salad and season with ground black pepper to taste.

This recipe is DASH diet•friendly because:

• Cucumbers and tomatoes are low•sodium, high•fiber vegetables that are rich in vitamins and minerals.

• Low•fat feta cheese provides a source of protein and calcium without excessive saturated fat or sodium.

• The red wine vinegar and olive oil dressing adds flavor without the need for added salt.

This recipe is also suitable for renal health because:

• Cucumbers, tomatoes, and low•fat feta cheese are all relatively low in potassium, making this a good choice for those with kidney disease.

• The overall sodium content is low, which is important for managing blood pressure and kidney function.

• The combination of fiber, protein, and healthy fats can help support overall nutrition and health.

23. Kale and Apple Salad with Lemon Dressing

Ingredient:

- 2 cups chopped kale, stems removed
- 1 medium apple, diced
- 2 tbsp chopped walnuts
- 1 tbsp lemon juice
- 1 tsp extra•virgin olive oil
- Ground black pepper to taste

Instructions:

1. In a large salad bowl, combine the chopped kale, diced apple, and chopped walnuts.

2. In a small bowl, whisk together the lemon juice and olive oil to make the dressing.

3. Drizzle the lemon dressing over the kale salad and toss gently to coat.

4. Season with ground black pepper to taste.

This recipe is DASH diet•friendly because:

- Kale is a low•sodium, high•fiber, and nutrient•dense green.

- Apples provide natural sweetness and fiber without added sugars.

- Walnuts are a source of healthy fats and protein without excessive sodium.

- The lemon juice and olive oil dressing adds flavor without the need for added salt.

This recipe is also suitable for renal health because:

- Kale, apples, and walnuts are all relatively low in potassium, making this a good choice for those with kidney disease.

- The overall sodium content is low, which is important for managing blood pressure and kidney function.

- The combination of fiber, healthy fats, and nutrients can help support overall nutrition and health.

24. Quinoa and Black Bean Salad

Ingredient:

- 1 cup cooked quinoa, cooled
- 1 (15 oz) can low•sodium black beans, rinsed and drained
- 1 cup diced bell pepper (any color)
- 1/2 cup diced red onion
- 2 tbsp chopped fresh cilantro
- 2 tbsp lime juice
- 1 tbsp extra•virgin olive oil
- 1/4 tsp ground cumin
- Salt and pepper to taste

Instructions:

1. In a large bowl, combine the cooked quinoa, black beans, diced bell pepper, red onion, and chopped cilantro.

2. In a small bowl, whisk together the lime juice, olive oil, and cumin.

3. Drizzle the dressing over the quinoa and bean mixture and toss gently to coat.

4. Season with salt and pepper to taste.

This recipe is DASH diet•friendly because:
- Quinoa is a whole grain that is high in fiber and protein.

- Black beans are a low•sodium, high•fiber, and high•protein legume.

- The bell pepper, onion, and cilantro provide additional vitamins, minerals, and antioxidants without excessive sodium. The lime juice and olive oil dressing adds flavor without the need for added salt.

This recipe is also suitable for renal health because:
- Quinoa, black beans, and the vegetables used are all relatively low in potassium, making this a good choice for those with kidney disease.

- The overall sodium content is low, which is important for managing blood pressure and kidney function.

- The combination of fiber, protein, and complex carbohydrates can help support overall nutrition and health.

25. Mixed Greens with Blueberries and Almonds

Ingredient:

• 4 cups mixed greens (such as spinach, arugula, and kale)
• 1/2 cup fresh blueberries
• 2 tbsp sliced almonds
• 1 tbsp balsamic vinegar
• 1 tsp extra•virgin olive oil
• Ground black pepper to taste

Instructions:

1. In a large salad bowl, combine the mixed greens, fresh blueberries, and sliced almonds.

2. In a small bowl, whisk together the balsamic vinegar and olive oil to make the dressing.

3. Drizzle the balsamic vinaigrette over the salad and toss gently to coat.

4. Season with ground black pepper to taste.

This recipe is DASH diet•friendly because:

• The mixed greens are low in sodium and high in fiber, vitamins, and minerals.

• Blueberries provide natural sweetness and antioxidants without added sugars.

• Almonds are a source of healthy fats and protein without excessive sodium.

• The balsamic vinegar and olive oil dressing adds flavor without the need for added salt.

This recipe is also suitable for renal health because:

• The mixed greens, blueberries, and almonds are all relatively low in potassium, making this a good choice for those with kidney disease.

• The overall sodium content is low, which is important for managing blood pressure and kidney function.

• The combination of fiber, healthy fats, and nutrients can help support overall nutrition and health.

26. Arugula Salad with Pears and Pecans

Ingredient:

• 4 cups arugula, washed and dried
• 1 medium pear, sliced
• 2 tbsp chopped pecans
• 1 tbsp balsamic vinegar
• 1 tsp extra•virgin olive oil
• Ground black pepper to taste

Instructions:

1. In a large salad bowl, combine the arugula, sliced pear, and chopped pecans.

2. In a small bowl, whisk together the balsamic vinegar and olive oil to make the dressing.

3. Drizzle the balsamic vinaigrette over the salad and toss gently to coat.

4. Season with ground black pepper to taste.

This recipe is DASH diet•friendly because:

• Arugula is a low•sodium, high•fiber, and nutrient•dense green.

• Pears provide natural sweetness and fiber without added sugars.

• Pecans are a source of healthy fats and protein without excessive sodium.

• The balsamic vinegar and olive oil dressing adds flavor without the need for added salt.

This recipe is also suitable for renal health because:

• Arugula, pears, and pecans are all relatively low in potassium, making this a good choice for those with kidney disease.

• The overall sodium content is low, which is important for managing blood pressure and kidney function.

• The combination of fiber, healthy fats, and nutrients can help support overall nutrition and health.

27. Chickpea Salad with Bell Peppers and Red Onion

Ingredient:

• 1 (15 oz) can low•sodium chickpeas, rinsed and drained
• 1/2 cup diced bell pepper (any color)
• 1/4 cup diced red onion
• 2 tbsp chopped fresh parsley
• 1 tbsp lemon juice
• 1 tsp extra•virgin olive oil
• 1/4 tsp ground cumin
• Salt and pepper to taste

Instructions:

1. In a medium bowl, combine the rinsed and drained chickpeas, diced bell pepper, diced red onion, and chopped parsley.

2. In a small bowl, whisk together the lemon juice, olive oil, and cumin to make the dressing.

3. Drizzle the dressing over the chickpea salad and toss gently to coat.

4. Season with salt and pepper to taste.

This recipe is DASH diet•friendly because:

• Chickpeas are a low•sodium, high•fiber, and high•protein legume.

• Bell peppers and red onion provide additional vitamins, minerals, and antioxidants without excessive sodium.

• The lemon juice and olive oil dressing adds flavor without the need for added salt.

This recipe is also suitable for renal health because:

• Chickpeas, bell peppers, and red onion are all relatively low in potassium, making this a good choice for those with kidney disease.

• The overall sodium content is low, which is important for managing blood pressure and kidney function.

• The combination of fiber, protein, and complex carbohydrates can help support overall nutrition and health.

28. Roasted Beet and Goat Cheese Salad

Ingredient:

• 2 medium beets, peeled and cut into 1•inch cubes
• 1 tbsp extra•virgin olive oil
• 4 cups mixed greens (such as spinach, arugula, and kale)
• 2 oz crumbled low•fat goat cheese
• 1 tbsp balsamic vinegar
• Ground black pepper to taste

Instructions:
1. Preheat the oven to 400°F. Toss the cubed beets with the olive oil and spread them on a baking sheet. Roast for 20•25 minutes, or until tender.

2. In a large salad bowl, combine the roasted beets and mixed greens.

3. Sprinkle the crumbled low•fat goat cheese over the salad.

4. In a small bowl, whisk together the balsamic vinegar.

5. Drizzle the balsamic vinegar over the salad and toss gently to coat. Season with ground black pepper to taste.

This recipe is DASH diet•friendly because:

• Beets are a low•sodium, high•fiber vegetable that is rich in vitamins and minerals.

• Low•fat goat cheese provides a source of protein and calcium without excessive saturated fat or sodium. The balsamic vinegar dressing adds flavor without the need for added salt.

This recipe is also suitable for renal health because:

• Beets and low•fat goat cheese are both relatively low in potassium, making this a good choice for those with kidney disease.

• The overall sodium content is low, which is important for managing blood pressure and kidney function.

• The combination of fiber, protein, and nutrients can help support overall nutrition and health.

29. Tomato, Cucumber, and Mint Salad

Ingredient:

• 2 cups diced tomatoes
• 1 cup diced cucumber
• 2 tbsp chopped fresh mint
• 1 tbsp red wine vinegar
• 1 tsp extra•virgin olive oil
• Ground black pepper to taste

Instructions:

1. In a medium bowl, combine the diced tomatoes, diced cucumber, and chopped fresh mint.

2. In a small bowl, whisk together the red wine vinegar and olive oil to make the dressing.

3. Drizzle the dressing over the salad and toss gently to coat.

4. Season with ground black pepper to taste.

This recipe is DASH diet•friendly because:

• Tomatoes and cucumbers are low•sodium, high•fiber vegetables that are rich in vitamins and minerals.

• Fresh mint adds flavor without the need for added salt.

• The red wine vinegar and olive oil dressing adds flavor without excessive sodium.

This recipe is also suitable for renal health because:

• Tomatoes, cucumbers, and mint are all relatively low in potassium, making this a good choice for those with kidney disease.

• The overall sodium content is low, which is important for managing blood pressure and kidney function.

• The combination of fiber, vitamins, and antioxidants can help support overall nutrition and health.

30. Lentil Salad with Carrots and Celery

Ingredient:

- 1 cup cooked lentils, cooled
- 1/2 cup diced carrots
- 1/2 cup diced celery
- 2 tbsp chopped fresh parsley
- 1 tbsp lemon juice
- 1 tsp extra•virgin olive oil
- 1/4 tsp ground cumin
- Salt and pepper to taste

Instructions:

1. In a medium bowl, combine the cooked and cooled lentils, diced carrots, diced celery, and chopped parsley.

2. In a small bowl, whisk together the lemon juice, olive oil, and cumin to make the dressing.

3. Drizzle the dressing over the lentil salad and toss gently to coat. Season with salt and pepper to taste.

This recipe is DASH diet•friendly because:

- Lentils are a low•sodium, high•fiber, and high•protein legume.

- Carrots and celery provide additional vitamins, minerals, and fiber without excessive sodium.

- The lemon juice and olive oil dressing adds flavor without the need for added salt.

This recipe is also suitable for renal health because:

- Lentils, carrots, and celery are all relatively low in potassium, making this a good choice for those with kidney disease.

- The overall sodium content is low, which is important for managing blood pressure and kidney function.

- The combination of fiber, protein, and complex carbohydrates can help support overall nutrition and health.

31. Low•Sodium Chicken and Vegetable Soup

Ingredient:

• 4 cups low•sodium chicken broth
• 1 boneless, skinless chicken breast, diced
• 1 cup diced carrots
• 1 cup diced celery
• 1 cup diced zucchini
• 1/2 cup diced onion
• 2 cloves garlic, minced
• 1 tsp dried thyme
• Ground black pepper to taste

Instructions:
1. In a large pot, combine the low•sodium chicken broth, diced chicken, carrots, celery, zucchini, onion, and garlic.

2. Bring the mixture to a boil over high heat, then reduce the heat and let it simmer for 15•20 minutes, or until the vegetables are tender and the chicken is cooked through.

3. Stir in the dried thyme and season with ground black pepper to taste.

This recipe is DASH diet•friendly because:
• It uses low•sodium chicken broth as the base, which reduces the overall sodium content.

• The variety of vegetables provides fiber, vitamins, and minerals without excessive sodium.

• The chicken breast is a lean protein source. The herbs and spices add flavor without the need for added salt.

This recipe is also suitable for renal health because:
• The vegetables used are relatively low in potassium, making this a good choice for those with kidney disease.

• The overall sodium content is low, which is important for managing blood pressure and kidney function.

• The protein, fiber, and nutrients in this soup can help support overall nutrition and health

32. Lentil Soup with Spinach

Ingredient:

- 1 cup dry brown or green lentils, rinsed
- 4 cups low•sodium vegetable or chicken broth
- 1 cup diced onion
- 1 cup diced carrots
- 1 cup diced celery
- 2 cloves garlic, minced
- 2 cups fresh spinach, chopped
- 1 tsp dried thyme
- 1/4 tsp ground black pepper
- Salt to taste (optional)

Instructions:

1. In a large pot, combine the rinsed lentils and broth. Bring to a boil over high heat.

2. Reduce heat to medium•low, cover, and simmer for 15•20 minutes, or until the lentils are tender.

3. Add the diced onion, carrots, celery, and garlic. Simmer for an additional 10 minutes.

4. Stir in the chopped spinach and dried thyme. Cook for 2•3 minutes, until the spinach is wilted. Season with ground black pepper and salt to taste, if desired.

This recipe is DASH diet•friendly because:
- Lentils are a low•sodium, high•fiber, and high•protein legume.

- The vegetables provide additional vitamins, minerals, and fiber without excessive sodium. The low•sodium broth and minimal added salt keep the overall sodium content low.

This recipe is also suitable for renal health because:
- Lentils, spinach, and the other vegetables are relatively low in potassium, making this a good choice for those with kidney disease.

- The overall sodium content is low, which is important for managing blood pressure and kidney function.

- The combination of protein, fiber, and nutrients can help support overall nutrition and health.

33. Butternut Squash Soup

Ingredient:

- 1 medium butternut squash, peeled, seeded, and cubed (about 4 cups)
- 1 medium onion, diced
- 2 cloves garlic, minced
- 4 cups low•sodium vegetable or chicken broth
- 1 tsp ground cinnamon
- 1/4 tsp ground nutmeg
- Ground black pepper to taste
- Chopped fresh parsley for garnish (optional)

Instructions:

1. In a large pot or Dutch oven, combine the cubed butternut squash, diced onion, and minced garlic.

2. Add the low•sodium broth and bring the mixture to a boil over high heat.

3. Reduce the heat to medium•low, cover, and simmer for 20•25 minutes, or until the squash is very soft.

4. Using an immersion blender or regular blender, puree the soup until smooth.

5. Stir in the ground cinnamon and nutmeg. Season with ground black pepper to taste. Serve the soup warm, garnished with chopped fresh parsley if desired.

This recipe is DASH diet•friendly because:
- Butternut squash is a low•sodium, high•fiber, and nutrient•dense vegetable. The onion and garlic provide additional flavor without the need for added salt.

- The low•sodium broth keeps the overall sodium content low.The spices add flavor without excessive sodium.

This recipe is also suitable for renal health because:
- Butternut squash is relatively low in potassium, making this a good choice for those with kidney disease.

- The overall sodium content is low, which is important for managing blood pressure and kidney function.

- The fiber, vitamins, and antioxidants in the squash can help support overall nutrition and health.

34. Tomato Basil Soup

Ingredient:
- 1 (28 oz) can low•sodium diced tomatoes
- 1 cup low•sodium vegetable or chicken broth
- 1/2 cup diced onion
- 2 cloves garlic, minced
- 1/4 cup chopped fresh basil
- 1 tsp dried oregano
- Ground black pepper to taste
- Pinch of red pepper flakes (optional)

Instructions:
1. In a medium saucepan, combine the low•sodium diced tomatoes, vegetable or chicken broth, diced onion, and minced garlic.

2. Bring the mixture to a simmer over medium heat, then reduce the heat and let it simmer for 10•15 minutes, stirring occasionally.

3. Remove the saucepan from the heat and stir in the chopped fresh basil and dried oregano.

4. Using an immersion blender or regular blender, puree the soup until smooth.

5. Season with ground black pepper and a pinch of red pepper flakes (if using) to taste.

This recipe is DASH diet•friendly because:
- It uses low•sodium canned tomatoes and broth to keep the overall sodium content low.

- The fresh basil and dried oregano add flavor without the need for added salt.

- The onion and garlic provide additional flavor without excessive sodium.

This recipe is also suitable for renal health because:
- Tomatoes, onions, and garlic are all relatively low in potassium, making this a good choice for those with kidney disease.

- The overall sodium content is low, which is important for managing blood pressure and kidney function.

- The fiber, vitamins, and antioxidants in the tomatoes can help support overall nutrition and health.

35. Broccoli and Cauliflower Soup

Ingredient:

- 1 tbsp olive oil
- 1 onion, diced
- 3 cloves garlic, minced
- 4 cups low•sodium vegetable or chicken broth
- 2 cups chopped broccoli florets
- 2 cups chopped cauliflower florets
- 1 tsp dried thyme
- 1/4 tsp ground black pepper
- 1/4 cup unsweetened almond milk or low•fat milk

Instructions:

1. In a large pot, heat the olive oil over medium heat. Add the onion and garlic and sauté for 3•4 minutes until softened.

2. Add the broth, broccoli, cauliflower, thyme, and black pepper. Bring to a boil, then reduce heat and simmer for 15•20 minutes, until the vegetables are tender.

3. Using an immersion blender or regular blender, puree the soup until smooth.

4. Stir in the almond milk or low•fat milk and heat through, but do not boil.

5. Serve hot.

This soup is low in sodium, high in fiber, and provides a good source of vitamins and minerals, making it a great option for those following a DASH diet or managing renal health. The broccoli and cauliflower provide antioxidants and anti•inflammatory benefits as well.

36. Carrot and Ginger Soup

Ingredient:

• 1 tbsp olive oil
• 1 onion, diced
• 3 cloves garlic, minced
• 1 tbsp grated fresh ginger
• 1 lb carrots, peeled and chopped
• 4 cups low•sodium vegetable or chicken broth
• 1 tsp ground cumin
• 1/4 tsp ground black pepper
• 1/4 cup unsweetened almond milk or low•fat milk

Instructions:

1. In a large pot, heat the olive oil over medium heat. Add the onion, garlic, and ginger, and sauté for 3•4 minutes until fragrant.

2. Add the chopped carrots, broth, cumin, and black pepper. Bring to a boil, then reduce heat and simmer for 20•25 minutes, until the carrots are very tender.

3. Using an immersion blender or regular blender, puree the soup until smooth.

4. Stir in the almond milk or low•fat milk and heat through, but do not boil.

5. Serve hot.

This soup is low in sodium, high in fiber, and provides a good source of vitamins and minerals, making it a great option for those following a DASH diet or managing renal health. The carrots and ginger provide anti•inflammatory benefits and support digestive health.

37. Minestrone Soup with Beans and Vegetables

Ingredient:

- 1 tbsp olive oil
- 1 onion, diced
- 3 cloves garlic, minced
- 2 carrots, peeled and diced
- 2 stalks celery, diced
- 1 zucchini, diced
- 1 can (15 oz) low•sodium diced tomatoes
- 4 cups low•sodium vegetable or chicken broth
- 1 can (15 oz) low•sodium kidney beans, rinsed and drained
- 1 cup frozen green beans
- 1 tsp dried oregano
- 1 tsp dried basil
- 1/4 tsp ground black pepper
- 2 cups cooked whole wheat pasta (optional)

Instructions:

1. In a large pot, heat the olive oil over medium heat. Add the onion and garlic and sauté for 3•4 minutes until fragrant.

2. Add the carrots, celery, and zucchini, and sauté for an additional 5 minutes.

3. Stir in the diced tomatoes, broth, kidney beans, green beans, oregano, basil, and black pepper. Bring to a boil, then reduce heat and simmer for 20•25 minutes, until the vegetables are tender.

4. If using, stir in the cooked whole wheat pasta and heat through.

5. Serve hot.

This minestrone soup is packed with fiber, vitamins, and minerals from the variety of vegetables and beans. It's low in sodium and suitable for those following a DASH diet or managing renal health. The whole wheat pasta adds extra fiber and complex carbohydrates.

38. Cabbage Soup with Ground Turkey

Ingredient:

• 1 lb ground turkey
• 1 tbsp olive oil
• 1 onion, diced
• 3 cloves garlic, minced
• 1 head green cabbage, chopped
• 4 cups low•sodium chicken or vegetable broth
• 1 can (15 oz) diced tomatoes
• 1 tsp dried oregano
• 1 tsp dried basil
• 1/4 tsp ground black pepper
• 1/4 tsp crushed red pepper flakes (optional)

Instructions:

1. In a large pot or Dutch oven, cook the ground turkey over medium•high heat until browned and cooked through, 5•7 minutes. Transfer the cooked turkey to a plate and set aside.

2. In the same pot, heat the olive oil over medium heat. Add the onion and garlic and sauté for 3•4 minutes until fragrant.

3. Add the chopped cabbage to the pot and sauté for 5•7 minutes, until the cabbage starts to soften.

4. Pour in the broth and diced tomatoes. Stir in the oregano, basil, black pepper, and red pepper flakes (if using).

5. Return the cooked ground turkey to the pot and bring the soup to a boil. Reduce heat and simmer for 20•25 minutes, until the cabbage is tender.

6. Serve hot.

This cabbage soup is a hearty and flavorful option that's high in protein from the ground turkey and fiber from the cabbage. It's a great meal for those looking for a comforting and nutritious soup.

39. Sweet Potato and Black Bean Soup

Ingredient:

- 1 tbsp olive oil
- 1 onion, diced
- 3 cloves garlic, minced
- 2 medium sweet potatoes, peeled and diced
- 1 can (15 oz) low•sodium black beans, rinsed and drained
- 4 cups low•sodium vegetable or chicken broth
- 1 tsp ground cumin
- 1 tsp chili powder
- 1/4 tsp ground black pepper
- 1/4 cup unsweetened almond milk or low•fat milk
- Chopped fresh cilantro for garnish (optional)

Instructions:

1. In a large pot, heat the olive oil over medium heat. Add the onion and garlic and sauté for 3•4 minutes until fragrant.

2. Add the diced sweet potatoes, black beans, broth, cumin, chili powder, and black pepper. Bring to a boil, then reduce heat and simmer for 20•25 minutes, until the sweet potatoes are tender.

3. Using an immersion blender or regular blender, puree the soup until smooth.

4. Stir in the almond milk or low•fat milk and heat through, but do not boil.

5. Serve hot, garnished with chopped fresh cilantro if desired.

This sweet potato and black bean soup is a nutritious and flavorful option that's high in fiber, vitamins, and minerals. The sweet potatoes provide a natural sweetness, while the black beans add protein and heartiness. It's a great option for a comforting and healthy meal.

40. Zucchini and Basil Soup

Ingredient:

- 1 tbsp olive oil
- 1 onion, diced
- 3 cloves garlic, minced
- 3 medium zucchini, chopped
- 4 cups low•sodium vegetable or chicken broth
- 1/2 cup fresh basil leaves, chopped
- 1 tsp dried oregano
- 1/4 tsp ground black pepper
- 1/4 cup unsweetened almond milk or low•fat milk

Instructions:

1. In a large pot, heat the olive oil over medium heat. Add the onion and garlic and sauté for 3•4 minutes until fragrant.

2. Add the chopped zucchini and broth to the pot. Bring to a boil, then reduce heat and simmer for 15•20 minutes, until the zucchini is very tender.

3. Using an immersion blender or regular blender, puree the soup until smooth.

4. Stir in the chopped basil, oregano, and black pepper.

5. Slowly stir in the almond milk or low•fat milk and heat through, but do not boil.

6. Serve hot.

This zucchini and basil soup is low in sodium, high in fiber, and provides a good source of vitamins and minerals, making it a great option for those following a DASH diet or managing renal health. The zucchini and basil provide anti•inflammatory benefits and support overall health.

41. Grilled Salmon with Asparagus

Ingredient:

• 4 (4 oz) salmon fillets
• 1 tbsp olive oil
• 1 tsp lemon zest
• 1 tbsp lemon juice
• 1 tsp dried dill
• 1/4 tsp ground black pepper
• 1 lb asparagus, trimmed
• 1 tbsp balsamic vinegar

Instructions:

1. Preheat grill or grill pan to medium•high heat.

2. In a small bowl, mix together the olive oil, lemon zest, lemon juice, dill, and black pepper. Brush the salmon fillets with the mixture on both sides.

3. Grill the salmon for 4•6 minutes per side, or until it flakes easily with a fork.

4. In a separate grill basket or on a grill•safe baking sheet, grill the asparagus for 5•7 minutes, turning occasionally, until tender•crisp.

5. Transfer the grilled salmon and asparagus to a serving plate. Drizzle the asparagus with the balsamic vinegar.

6. Serve immediately.

This grilled salmon and asparagus dish is a great option for those following a DASH diet or managing renal health. Salmon is a heart•healthy source of protein and omega•3 fatty acids, while asparagus is low in sodium and high in fiber, vitamins, and minerals. The lemon, dill, and balsamic vinegar add flavor without the need for excessive sodium.

42. Baked Chicken Breast with Quinoa

Ingredient:

• 4 (4 oz) boneless, skinless chicken breasts
• 1 tbsp olive oil
• 1 tsp dried thyme
• 1/2 tsp garlic powder
• 1/4 tsp ground black pepper
• 1 cup uncooked quinoa, rinsed
• 2 cups low•sodium chicken or vegetable broth
• 1 cup chopped fresh spinach
• 1 tbsp lemon juice

Instructions:

1. Preheat oven to 400°F.

2. Place the chicken breasts in a baking dish and brush with the olive oil. Sprinkle with the thyme, garlic powder, and black pepper.

3. Bake the chicken for 25•30 minutes, or until it reaches an internal temperature of 165°F.

4. While the chicken is baking, combine the quinoa and broth in a saucepan. Bring to a boil, then reduce heat and simmer for 15•20 minutes, until the quinoa is tender and the liquid is absorbed.

5. Fluff the cooked quinoa with a fork and stir in the chopped spinach and lemon juice.

6. Serve the baked chicken breast on top of the quinoa and spinach mixture.

This baked chicken and quinoa dish is a great option for those following a DASH diet or managing renal health. The chicken provides lean protein, while the quinoa is a whole grain that's high in fiber and nutrients. The spinach adds additional vitamins and minerals, and the lemon juice provides a bright, fresh flavor without the need for excessive sodium.

43. Turkey Meatballs with Whole Grain Pasta

Ingredient:

- 1 lb ground turkey
- 1/2 cup whole wheat breadcrumbs
- 1/4 cup grated Parmesan cheese
- 1 egg, lightly beaten
- 2 cloves garlic, minced
- 1 tsp dried oregano
- 1/4 tsp ground black pepper
- 8 oz whole grain pasta (such as whole wheat or brown rice pasta)
- 1 jar (24 oz) low•sodium marinara sauce
- 2 cups fresh spinach, chopped

Instructions:

1. Preheat oven to 400°F. Line a baking sheet with parchment paper.

2. In a large bowl, combine the ground turkey, breadcrumbs, Parmesan, egg, garlic, oregano, and black pepper. Mix well until fully incorporated.

3. Roll the mixture into 1•inch meatballs and place them on the prepared baking sheet.

4. Bake the meatballs for 18•20 minutes, or until cooked through.

5. While the meatballs are baking, cook the whole grain pasta according to package instructions. Drain and set aside.

6. In a large saucepan, heat the low•sodium marinara sauce over medium heat. Add the cooked meatballs and chopped spinach to the sauce and simmer for 5 minutes.

7. Serve the meatballs and sauce over the cooked whole grain pasta.

This turkey meatball and whole grain pasta dish is a great option for those following a DASH diet or managing renal health. The turkey provides lean protein, the whole grain pasta is high in fiber, and the spinach adds additional vitamins and minerals. The low•sodium marinara sauce keeps the sodium content in check.

44. Tofu Stir•Fry with Mixed Vegetables

Ingredient:

• 1 block (14 oz) extra•firm tofu, drained and cubed
• 1 tbsp sesame oil
• 2 cloves garlic, minced
• 1 tbsp grated fresh ginger
• 1 red bell pepper, sliced
• 1 cup broccoli florets
• 1 cup snow peas
• 1 cup sliced mushrooms
• 2 cups baby spinach
• 2 tbsp low•sodium soy sauce or tamari
• 1 tbsp rice vinegar
• 1 tsp sesame seeds (optional)

Instructions:

1. Heat the sesame oil in a large wok or skillet over medium•high heat.

2. Add the cubed tofu and stir•fry for 3•4 minutes, until lightly browned. Transfer the tofu to a plate and set aside.

3. In the same wok or skillet, add the garlic and ginger and stir•fry for 1 minute until fragrant.

4. Add the sliced bell pepper, broccoli, snow peas, and mushrooms. Stir•fry for 5•7 minutes, until the vegetables are tender•crisp.

5. Add the spinach and stir•fry for 1•2 minutes, until the spinach is wilted.

6. Return the cooked tofu to the wok or skillet. Stir in the soy sauce or tamari and rice vinegar. Toss everything together until well combined.

7. Serve the tofu stir•fry hot, garnished with sesame seeds if desired.

This tofu stir•fry is a great option for those following a DASH diet or managing renal health. Tofu is a plant•based protein source, and the mixed vegetables provide a variety of vitamins, minerals, and fiber. The low•sodium soy sauce or tamari keeps the sodium content in check.

45. Shrimp and Broccoli Stir•Fry

Ingredient:

• 1 lb peeled and deveined shrimp
• 2 tbsp low•sodium soy sauce or tamari
• 1 tbsp rice vinegar
• 1 tsp sesame oil
• 1 tbsp olive oil
• 3 cloves garlic, minced
• 1 tbsp grated fresh ginger
• 4 cups broccoli florets
• 1 red bell pepper, sliced
• 1/4 cup low•sodium chicken or vegetable broth
• 1 tsp cornstarch
• 2 cups cooked brown rice

Instructions:

1. In a small bowl, combine the soy sauce or tamari, rice vinegar, and sesame oil. Set aside.

2. Heat the olive oil in a large wok or skillet over medium•high heat. Add the garlic and ginger and stir•fry for 1 minute until fragrant.

3. Add the shrimp and stir•fry for 2•3 minutes, until the shrimp start to turn pink.

4. Add the broccoli florets and bell pepper slices. Stir•fry for 3•4 minutes, until the vegetables are tender•crisp.

5. In a small bowl, whisk together the broth and cornstarch. Pour the mixture into the wok or skillet and stir to coat the shrimp and vegetables.

6. Stir in the soy sauce mixture and cook for 1•2 minutes, until the sauce has thickened slightly.

7. Serve the shrimp and broccoli stir•fry over the cooked brown rice.

This shrimp and broccoli stir•fry is a great option for those following a DASH diet or managing renal health. Shrimp is a lean protein source, and the broccoli and bell pepper provide fiber, vitamins, and minerals. The low•sodium soy sauce or tamari and broth keep the sodium content in check.

46. Black Bean and Sweet Potato Tacos

Ingredient:

- 2 medium sweet potatoes, peeled and diced
- 1 tbsp olive oil
- 1 tsp ground cumin
- 1/4 tsp chili powder
- 1/4 tsp ground black pepper
- 1 can (15 oz) low·sodium black beans, rinsed and drained
- 1/4 cup low·sodium vegetable broth
- 8 small whole wheat tortillas or taco shells
- 1 cup shredded green cabbage
- 1/4 cup chopped fresh cilantro
- 1 avocado, sliced (optional)
- Lime wedges for serving

Instructions:

1. Preheat oven to 400°F. Toss the diced sweet potatoes with the olive oil, cumin, chili powder, and black pepper. Spread on a baking sheet and roast for 20·25 minutes, until tender.

2. In a medium saucepan, combine the black beans and vegetable broth. Heat over medium heat, stirring occasionally, until heated through.

3. To assemble the tacos, place a spoonful of the roasted sweet potatoes and black beans in each tortilla or taco shell. Top with shredded cabbage, chopped cilantro, and avocado slices (if using).

4. Serve the tacos with lime wedges on the side.

These black bean and sweet potato tacos are a great option for those following a DASH diet or managing renal health. The sweet potatoes and black beans provide fiber, vitamins, and minerals, while the whole wheat tortillas or taco shells are a whole grain option. The low·sodium broth and lack of added salt keep the sodium content in check.

47. Lemon Herb Baked Tilapia

Ingredient:

- 4 (4 oz) tilapia fillets
- 1 tbsp olive oil
- 2 tbsp lemon juice
- 1 tsp dried parsley
- 1 tsp dried dill
- 1/2 tsp garlic powder
- 1/4 tsp ground black pepper
- 1 lemon, sliced (for serving)

Instructions:

1. Preheat oven to 400°F. Lightly grease a baking dish or line it with parchment paper.

2. Place the tilapia fillets in the prepared baking dish.

3. In a small bowl, whisk together the olive oil, lemon juice, parsley, dill, garlic powder, and black pepper.

4. Drizzle the lemon•herb mixture over the tilapia fillets, making sure to evenly coat the fish.

5. Bake for 15•18 minutes, or until the fish flakes easily with a fork and reaches an internal temperature of 145°F.

6. Serve the baked tilapia immediately, garnished with lemon slices.

This lemon herb baked tilapia is a great option for those following a DASH diet or managing renal health. Tilapia is a lean, mild•flavored fish that's high in protein and low in mercury. The lemon, herbs, and spices add flavor without the need for excessive sodium. Serve it with a side of steamed vegetables or a fresh salad for a complete and healthy meal.

48. Spaghetti Squash with Tomato Sauce

Ingredient:

• 1 medium spaghetti squash, halved lengthwise and seeded
• 1 tbsp olive oil
• 1 onion, diced
• 3 cloves garlic, minced
• 1 can (28 oz) low•sodium diced tomatoes
• 2 tbsp fresh basil, chopped
• 1 tsp dried oregano
• 1/4 tsp ground black pepper
• 1/4 cup grated Parmesan cheese (optional)

Instructions:

1. Preheat oven to 400°F. Place the spaghetti squash halves cut•side down on a baking sheet. Bake for 40•50 minutes, until the squash is tender and easily shreds with a fork.

2. In a large skillet, heat the olive oil over medium heat. Add the diced onion and sauté for 3•4 minutes until translucent.

3. Add the minced garlic and sauté for an additional minute until fragrant.

4. Pour in the can of low•sodium diced tomatoes, including the juice. Stir in the chopped basil, dried oregano, and black pepper.

5. Simmer the tomato sauce for 10•15 minutes, stirring occasionally, until slightly thickened.

6. Use a fork to shred the cooked spaghetti squash into strands. Transfer the squash strands to a serving dish.

7. Pour the tomato sauce over the spaghetti squash and toss to combine.

8. Serve the spaghetti squash with tomato sauce, optionally topped with a sprinkle of grated Parmesan cheese.

This spaghetti squash with tomato sauce dish is a great option for those following a DASH diet or managing renal health. Spaghetti squash is a low•calorie, low•carb alternative to traditional pasta, and the tomato sauce is low in sodium and high in vitamins and antioxidants.

49. Grilled Portobello Mushrooms

Ingredient:

- 4 large portobello mushroom caps, stems removed
- 2 tbsp olive oil
- 2 tbsp balsamic vinegar
- 2 cloves garlic, minced
- 1 tsp dried thyme
- 1/4 tsp ground black pepper

Instructions:

1. Preheat grill or grill pan to medium•high heat.

2. In a shallow dish, whisk together the olive oil, balsamic vinegar, garlic, thyme, and black pepper.

3. Add the portobello mushroom caps to the dish and turn to coat both sides with the marinade.

4. Grill the mushrooms for 4•5 minutes per side, or until they are tender and have grill marks.

5. Transfer the grilled portobello mushrooms to a serving plate.

Serve the grilled portobello mushrooms as a main dish, or use them as a vegetarian burger patty or topping for salads and sandwiches.

These grilled portobello mushrooms are a great option for a meatless, flavorful meal. The balsamic vinegar and herbs add depth of flavor without the need for excessive sodium or fat. Portobello mushrooms are a good source of fiber, vitamins, and minerals, making this a nutritious and satisfying dish.

50. Stuffed Bell Peppers with Ground Turkey

Ingredient:

• 4 large bell peppers (any color), halved lengthwise and seeded
• 1 lb ground turkey
• 1 cup cooked brown rice
• 1 onion, diced
• 2 cloves garlic, minced
• 1 can (15 oz) low•sodium diced tomatoes
• 1 tsp dried oregano
• 1/4 tsp ground black pepper
• 1/4 cup low•sodium chicken or vegetable broth
• 1/4 cup shredded low•fat mozzarella cheese (optional)

Instructions:

1. Preheat oven to 375°F.

2. Place the bell pepper halves in a baking dish and set aside.

3. In a large skillet, cook the ground turkey over medium heat until browned and crumbled, about 5•7 minutes. Drain any excess fat.

4. Add the diced onion and minced garlic to the skillet and sauté for 2•3 minutes until fragrant.

5. Stir in the cooked brown rice, diced tomatoes, oregano, and black pepper. Cook for an additional 2•3 minutes.

6. Spoon the turkey and rice mixture into the bell pepper halves, packing it in gently.

7. Pour the broth into the bottom of the baking dish, being careful not to pour it over the stuffed peppers.

8. Cover the dish with foil and bake for 30•35 minutes, or until the peppers are tender.

9. If desired, remove the foil and sprinkle the tops of the stuffed peppers with the shredded mozzarella cheese. Bake for an additional 5 minutes, or until the cheese is melted. Serve the stuffed bell peppers hot.

This stuffed bell pepper dish is a great option for those following a DASH diet or managing renal health. The ground turkey provides lean protein, the brown rice is a whole grain, and the bell peppers are low in sodium and high in vitamins and fiber.

51. Chickpea and Spinach Curry

Ingredient:

- 1 tbsp olive oil
- 1 onion, diced
- 3 cloves garlic, minced
- 1 tbsp grated fresh ginger
- 1 tsp ground cumin
- 1 tsp ground coriander
- 1 tsp garam masala
- 1/4 tsp ground cayenne pepper (optional)
- 1 can (15 oz) low•sodium chickpeas, rinsed and drained
- 1 can (14 oz) low•sodium diced tomatoes
- 1 cup low•sodium vegetable broth
- 4 cups fresh spinach, chopped
- 1/4 cup unsweetened almond milk or low•fat yogurt
- 1/4 tsp ground black pepper
- Chopped fresh cilantro for garnish (optional)

Instructions:

1. In a large skillet or saucepan, heat the olive oil over medium heat. Add the diced onion and sauté for 3•4 minutes until translucent.

2. Add the minced garlic and grated ginger to the skillet and sauté for 1 minute until fragrant.

3. Stir in the ground cumin, coriander, garam masala, and cayenne pepper (if using). Cook for 1 minute to toast the spices.

4. Add the rinsed and drained chickpeas, diced tomatoes, and vegetable broth. Bring the mixture to a simmer and cook for 10•15 minutes, until slightly thickened.

5. Stir in the chopped spinach and cook for 2•3 minutes, until the spinach is wilted.

6. Remove the curry from heat and stir in the almond milk or yogurt. Season with ground black pepper.

7. Serve the chickpea and spinach curry hot, garnished with chopped fresh cilantro if desired. Serve over cooked brown rice or quinoa, if desired.

This chickpea and spinach curry is a flavorful and nutritious dish that follows the DASH diet principles. Chickpeas provide plant•based protein, while the spinach and spices add fiber, vitamins, and anti•inflammatory benefits.

52. Lentil and Vegetable Stew

Ingredient:

- 1 tbsp olive oil
- 1 onion, diced
- 3 cloves garlic, minced
- 2 carrots, peeled and diced
- 2 stalks celery, diced
- 1 cup dried brown or green lentils, rinsed
- 4 cups low•sodium vegetable broth
- 1 can (15 oz) low•sodium diced tomatoes
- 2 cups chopped kale or spinach
- 1 tsp dried thyme
- 1 tsp dried oregano
- 1/4 tsp ground black pepper
- 1/4 cup unsweetened almond milk or low•fat milk (optional)

Instructions:

1. In a large pot or Dutch oven, heat the olive oil over medium heat. Add the diced onion and sauté for 3•4 minutes until translucent.

2. Add the minced garlic, diced carrots, and diced celery. Sauté for an additional 5 minutes.

3. Stir in the rinsed lentils, vegetable broth, diced tomatoes, chopped kale or spinach, thyme, oregano, and black pepper.

4. Bring the stew to a boil, then reduce heat and simmer for 25•30 minutes, or until the lentils are tender.

5. If desired, stir in the unsweetened almond milk or low•fat milk to add a creamy texture. Serve the lentil and vegetable stew hot.

This lentil and vegetable stew is a great option for those following a DASH diet or managing renal health. Lentils are a high•fiber, plant•based protein source, while the vegetables provide a variety of vitamins, minerals, and antioxidants. The low•sodium broth and lack of added salt keep the sodium content in check.

53. Quinoa Stuffed Zucchini Boats

Ingredient:

• 4 medium zucchini, halved lengthwise
• 1 cup cooked quinoa
• 1 can (15 oz) low•sodium black beans, rinsed and drained
• 1 cup diced tomatoes
• 1/2 cup crumbled feta cheese (optional)
• 2 tbsp chopped fresh basil
• 1 tsp dried oregano
• 1/4 tsp ground black pepper

Instructions:

1. Preheat oven to 400°F.

2. Scoop out the flesh from the zucchini halves, leaving about 1/4 inch of the zucchini shell. Chop the scooped•out zucchini flesh.

3. In a medium bowl, combine the chopped zucchini flesh, cooked quinoa, black beans, diced tomatoes, feta cheese (if using), basil, oregano, and black pepper. Mix well.

4. Spoon the quinoa mixture evenly into the zucchini boats, packing it in gently.

5. Place the stuffed zucchini boats in a baking dish. Cover with foil and bake for 25•30 minutes, or until the zucchini is tender.

6. Remove the foil and bake for an additional 5 minutes to lightly brown the tops.

7. Serve the quinoa stuffed zucchini boats warm.

These quinoa stuffed zucchini boats are a great option for those following a DASH diet or managing renal health. The zucchini provides fiber and nutrients, while the quinoa and black beans offer plant•based protein and complex carbohydrates. The feta cheese is optional, but it adds a nice tangy flavor.

54. Eggplant Parmesan (Baked)

Ingredient:

• 2 medium eggplants, sliced into 1/2•inch thick rounds
• 1 tbsp olive oil
• 1 cup whole wheat breadcrumbs
• 1/2 cup grated Parmesan cheese
• 1 tsp dried oregano
• 1/4 tsp ground black pepper
• 1 jar (24 oz) low•sodium marinara sauce
• 1 cup shredded part•skim mozzarella cheese

Instructions:
1. Preheat oven to 400°F. Lightly grease a baking sheet.

2. Arrange the eggplant slices in a single layer on the prepared baking sheet. Brush the tops of the eggplant slices with the olive oil.

3. In a shallow bowl, mix together the whole wheat breadcrumbs, Parmesan cheese, oregano, and black pepper.

4. Dip each eggplant slice into the breadcrumb mixture, coating both sides.

5. Place the breaded eggplant slices back on the baking sheet.

6. Bake for 20•25 minutes, flipping the slices halfway through, until the eggplant is tender and the breadcrumbs are golden brown.

7. Spread a thin layer of the low•sodium marinara sauce in the bottom of a baking dish. Arrange the baked eggplant slices in a single layer on top of the sauce.

8. Top the eggplant with the remaining marinara sauce and the shredded mozzarella cheese.

9. Bake for an additional 15•20 minutes, until the cheese is melted and bubbly. Let the eggplant parmesan cool for 5 minutes before serving.

This baked eggplant parmesan dish is a healthier version that follows the DASH diet principles. The eggplant provides fiber and nutrients, while the whole wheat breadcrumbs and low•sodium marinara sauce keep the sodium content in check.

55. Black Bean Burgers

Ingredient:

- 1 can (15 oz) low•sodium black beans, rinsed and drained
- 1/2 cup cooked quinoa
- 1/2 cup whole wheat breadcrumbs
- 1 egg, lightly beaten
- 2 tbsp chopped fresh cilantro
- 1 tsp ground cumin
- 1/4 tsp chili powder
- 1/4 tsp garlic powder
- 1/4 tsp ground black pepper
- 4 whole wheat hamburger buns
- Toppings (such as sliced avocado, tomato, lettuce, etc.)

Instructions:

1. In a large bowl, mash the black beans with a fork or potato masher, leaving some beans slightly chunky.

2. Add the cooked quinoa, whole wheat breadcrumbs, egg, cilantro, cumin, chili powder, garlic powder, and black pepper. Mix well until fully combined.

3. Divide the black bean mixture into 4 equal portions and shape them into patties, about 1/2 inch thick.

4. Heat a large non•stick skillet over medium heat. Cook the black bean patties for 4•5 minutes per side, or until lightly browned and heated through.

5. Serve the black bean burgers on the whole wheat buns, topped with your desired toppings.

These black bean burgers are a great option for those following a DASH diet or managing renal health. The black beans provide plant•based protein and fiber, while the whole wheat buns and breadcrumbs are a whole grain choice. The lack of added salt keeps the sodium content low.

56. Vegetable Paella

Ingredient:

- 1 tbsp olive oil
- 1 onion, diced
- 3 cloves garlic, minced
- 1 cup uncooked short•grain brown rice
- 1 tsp smoked paprika
- 1/2 tsp saffron threads (optional)
- 1/4 tsp ground black pepper
- 2 cups low•sodium vegetable broth
- 1 cup diced tomatoes
- 1 cup frozen peas
- 1 red bell pepper, diced
- 1 cup sliced mushrooms
- 1 cup chopped spinach
- 1/4 cup chopped fresh parsley

Instructions:

1. In a large skillet or paella pan, heat the olive oil over medium heat. Add the diced onion and sauté for 3•4 minutes until translucent.

2. Add the minced garlic and sauté for an additional minute until fragrant.

3. Stir in the uncooked brown rice, smoked paprika, saffron (if using), and black pepper. Cook for 2•3 minutes to toast the rice.

4. Pour in the low•sodium vegetable broth and add the diced tomatoes. Bring the mixture to a boil, then reduce heat and simmer for 20•25 minutes, until the rice is tender and has absorbed most of the liquid.

5. Stir in the frozen peas, diced bell pepper, sliced mushrooms, and chopped spinach. Cook for an additional 5•7 minutes, until the vegetables are tender.

6. Remove from heat and stir in the chopped fresh parsley. Serve the vegetable paella hot.

This vegetable paella is a flavorful and nutritious dish that follows the DASH diet principles. The brown rice, vegetables, and herbs provide a variety of vitamins, minerals, and antioxidants, while the low•sodium broth keeps the sodium content in check.

57. Cauliflower Fried Rice

Ingredient:

• 1 head of cauliflower, cut into florets
• 1 tbsp sesame oil
• 1 onion, diced
• 2 cloves garlic, minced
• 1 cup frozen peas and carrots
• 2 eggs, lightly beaten
• 2 tbsp low•sodium soy sauce or tamari
• 1 tsp sesame seeds (optional)
• 1/4 tsp ground black pepper

Instructions:

1. In a food processor, pulse the cauliflower florets until they resemble the size and texture of rice grains. Set aside.

2. Heat the sesame oil in a large skillet or wok over medium•high heat.

3. Add the diced onion and minced garlic to the skillet. Sauté for 2•3 minutes until fragrant.

4. Add the riced cauliflower and frozen peas and carrots to the skillet. Stir•fry for 5•7 minutes, until the cauliflower is tender.

5. Push the cauliflower mixture to the side of the skillet. Pour the lightly beaten eggs into the empty side and scramble them, then mix them into the cauliflower.

6. Stir in the low•sodium soy sauce or tamari and black pepper.

7. Serve the cauliflower fried rice hot, garnished with sesame seeds if desired.

This cauliflower fried rice is a great low•carb, low•sodium alternative to traditional fried rice. The cauliflower provides fiber and nutrients, while the soy sauce or tamari adds flavor without excessive sodium. It's a delicious and healthy option for those following a DASH diet or managing renal health.

58. Sweet Potato and Black Bean Enchiladas

Ingredient:

• 2 medium sweet potatoes, peeled and diced
• 1 tbsp olive oil
• 1 onion, diced
• 2 cloves garlic, minced
• 1 can (15 oz) low•sodium black beans, rinsed and drained
• 1 tsp ground cumin
• 1/2 tsp chili powder
• 1/4 tsp ground black pepper
• 8 whole wheat tortillas
• 1 can (15 oz) low•sodium enchilada sauce
• 1/2 cup shredded low•fat cheddar cheese

Instructions:
1. Preheat oven to 375°F.

2. In a large skillet, heat the olive oil over medium heat. Add the diced sweet potatoes and sauté for 8•10 minutes, until tender.

3. Add the diced onion and minced garlic to the skillet. Sauté for 3•4 minutes until the onion is translucent.

4. Stir in the rinsed and drained black beans, cumin, chili powder, and black pepper. Cook for 2•3 minutes to blend the flavors.

5. Spread 1/4 cup of the sweet potato and black bean mixture onto each whole wheat tortilla. Roll up the tortillas and place them seam•side down in a baking dish.

6. Pour the low•sodium enchilada sauce evenly over the enchiladas. Sprinkle the shredded cheddar cheese on top.

7. Bake for 20•25 minutes, until the cheese is melted and the enchiladas are heated through. Serve the sweet potato and black bean enchiladas hot.

These sweet potato and black bean enchiladas are a delicious and nutritious option that follows the DASH diet principles. The sweet potatoes, black beans, and whole wheat tortillas provide fiber, complex carbohydrates, and plant•based protein, while the low•sodium enchilada sauce keeps the sodium content in check.

59. Vegetable Stir•Fry with Brown Rice

Ingredient:

- 1 cup uncooked brown rice
- 1 tbsp sesame oil
- 1 onion, sliced
- 2 cloves garlic, minced
- 1 red bell pepper, sliced
- 1 cup broccoli florets
- 1 cup sliced mushrooms
- 1 cup snow peas
- 2 cups baby spinach
- 2 tbsp low•sodium soy sauce or tamari
- 1 tsp sesame seeds (optional)

Instructions:

1. Cook the brown rice according to package instructions.

2. In a large skillet or wok, heat the sesame oil over medium•high heat.

3. Add the sliced onion and minced garlic to the skillet. Sauté for 2•3 minutes until fragrant.

4. Add the sliced red bell pepper, broccoli florets, sliced mushrooms, and snow peas to the skillet. Stir•fry for 5•7 minutes, until the vegetables are tender•crisp.

5. Stir in the baby spinach and soy sauce or tamari. Cook for an additional 1•2 minutes, until the spinach is wilted.

6. Serve the vegetable stir•fry over the cooked brown rice, garnished with sesame seeds if desired.

This vegetable stir•fry with brown rice is a great option for those following a DASH diet or managing renal health. The brown rice provides complex carbohydrates and fiber, while the variety of vegetables offer a range of vitamins, minerals, and antioxidants. The low•sodium soy sauce or tamari keeps the sodium content in check.

60. Spinach and Ricotta Stuffed Shells

Ingredient:

- 12 jumbo pasta shells
- 1 cup part•skim ricotta cheese
- 1 cup chopped fresh spinach
- 1/4 cup grated Parmesan cheese
- 1 egg, lightly beaten
- 1/4 tsp ground black pepper
- 1 jar (24 oz) low•sodium marinara sauce
- 1/2 cup shredded part•skim mozzarella cheese

Instructions:

1. Preheat oven to 375°F.

2. Cook the pasta shells according to package instructions. Drain and set aside.

3. In a medium bowl, mix together the ricotta cheese, chopped spinach, Parmesan cheese, egg, and black pepper until well combined.

4. Spread 1/2 cup of the low•sodium marinara sauce in the bottom of a baking dish.

5. Stuff each cooked pasta shell with a heaping tablespoon of the ricotta•spinach mixture. Arrange the stuffed shells in the baking dish.

6. Pour the remaining marinara sauce over the stuffed shells, making sure to cover them completely.

7. Sprinkle the shredded mozzarella cheese over the top.

8. Bake for 25•30 minutes, until the cheese is melted and bubbly.

9. Let the stuffed shells cool for 5 minutes before serving.

These spinach and ricotta stuffed shells are a delicious and nutritious option that follows the DASH diet principles. The ricotta and Parmesan cheeses provide protein, while the spinach adds fiber and vitamins. The low•sodium marinara sauce keeps the sodium content in check.

61. Steamed Broccoli with Lemon

Ingredient:

- 1 lb broccoli florets
- 1 tbsp lemon juice
- 1 tsp olive oil
- 1/4 tsp garlic powder
- 1/4 tsp ground black pepper
- 1 tbsp chopped fresh parsley (optional)

Instructions:

1. Fill a large pot with 1•2 inches of water and bring to a boil.

2. Place the broccoli florets in a steamer basket and lower it into the pot. Cover and steam for 5•7 minutes, until the broccoli is tender•crisp.

3. Carefully remove the steamer basket from the pot and transfer the steamed broccoli to a serving bowl.

4. Drizzle the lemon juice and olive oil over the broccoli. Sprinkle with the garlic powder and ground black pepper. Toss gently to coat.

5. If desired, garnish the broccoli with chopped fresh parsley.

6. Serve the steamed broccoli with lemon warm or at room temperature.

This simple steamed broccoli dish is a great option for those following a DASH diet or managing renal health. Broccoli is low in sodium and high in fiber, vitamins, and minerals. The lemon juice, olive oil, and seasonings add flavor without the need for excessive sodium.

This side dish pairs well with grilled or baked proteins, such as chicken, fish, or tofu, for a complete and balanced meal.

62. Roasted Brussels Sprouts with Garlic

Ingredient:

• 1 lb Brussels sprouts, trimmed and halved
• 2 tbsp olive oil
• 3 cloves garlic, minced
• 1/4 tsp ground black pepper
• 1/8 tsp salt (optional)

Instructions:

1. Preheat oven to 400°F. Line a baking sheet with parchment paper.

2. In a large bowl, toss the trimmed and halved Brussels sprouts with the olive oil, minced garlic, black pepper, and salt (if using).

3. Spread the Brussels sprouts in a single layer on the prepared baking sheet.

4. Roast for 20•25 minutes, tossing halfway, until the Brussels sprouts are tender and lightly browned.

5. Serve the roasted Brussels sprouts with garlic hot.

This simple roasted Brussels sprouts dish is a great way to enjoy this nutritious vegetable. The garlic adds flavor, while the minimal seasoning allows the natural taste of the Brussels sprouts to shine.

Brussels sprouts are a great source of fiber, vitamins, and minerals. Roasting them brings out their natural sweetness and creates a delightful texture.

This dish can be served as a side or incorporated into other meals, such as salads or grain bowls. It's a versatile and healthy option that's easy to prepare.

63. Mashed Cauliflower

Ingredient:

• 1 large head of cauliflower, cut into florets
• 1/4 cup unsweetened almond milk or low•fat milk
• 2 tbsp olive oil
• 1 tsp garlic powder
• 1/4 tsp ground black pepper
• 1/8 tsp salt (optional)
• 2 tbsp chopped fresh chives (optional)

Instructions:

1. In a large pot, bring 1•2 inches of water to a boil. Add the cauliflower florets, cover, and steam for 10•12 minutes, until very tender.

2. Drain the cauliflower and transfer it to a food processor or high•powered blender.

3. Add the unsweetened almond milk or low•fat milk, olive oil, garlic powder, and black pepper. Season with a small amount of salt, if desired.

4. Blend or process the cauliflower mixture until smooth and creamy, scraping down the sides as needed.

5. Transfer the mashed cauliflower to a serving bowl and stir in the chopped fresh chives, if using.

6. Serve the mashed cauliflower warm.

This mashed cauliflower is a great low•carb, low•calorie alternative to traditional mashed potatoes. The cauliflower provides fiber, vitamins, and minerals, while the almond milk or low•fat milk adds creaminess without excessive fat or calories.

The garlic powder and black pepper provide flavor, and the optional chives add a fresh, herbal note. This mashed cauliflower can be enjoyed as a side dish or used as a base for other recipes.

64. Quinoa Pilaf with Vegetables

Ingredient:

- 1 cup uncooked quinoa, rinsed
- 2 cups low•sodium vegetable broth
- 1 tbsp olive oil
- 1 onion, diced
- 2 cloves garlic, minced
- 1 cup diced carrots
- 1 cup diced zucchini
- 1 cup diced bell pepper
- 1 cup frozen peas
- 2 tbsp chopped fresh parsley
- 1 tsp dried thyme
- 1/4 tsp ground black pepper

Instructions:

1. In a medium saucepan, combine the rinsed quinoa and vegetable broth. Bring to a boil, then reduce heat, cover, and simmer for 15•20 minutes, until the quinoa is tender and the liquid is absorbed.

2. In a large skillet, heat the olive oil over medium heat. Add the diced onion and minced garlic, and sauté for 3•4 minutes until fragrant.

3. Add the diced carrots, zucchini, and bell pepper to the skillet. Sauté for 5•7 minutes, until the vegetables are tender•crisp.

4. Stir the cooked quinoa, frozen peas, chopped parsley, dried thyme, and black pepper into the vegetable mixture. Cook for an additional 2•3 minutes, until everything is heated through.

5. Serve the quinoa pilaf with vegetables warm.

This quinoa pilaf is a great option for those following a DASH diet or managing renal health. Quinoa is a whole grain that's high in protein and fiber, while the variety of vegetables provide a range of vitamins, minerals, and antioxidants. The low•sodium vegetable broth keeps the sodium content in check.

65. Brown Rice with Herbs

Ingredient:

- 1 cup brown rice
- 2 cups vegetable or chicken broth
- 2 tablespoons olive oil
- 2 cloves garlic, minced
- 1 teaspoon dried thyme
- 1 teaspoon dried oregano
- 1/4 cup chopped fresh parsley
- Salt and pepper to taste

Instructions:

1. In a medium saucepan, bring the broth to a boil over high heat. Add the brown rice, cover, reduce heat to low and simmer for 45•50 minutes, until rice is tender and liquid is absorbed.

2. In a skillet, heat the olive oil over medium heat. Add the minced garlic and sauté for 1 minute until fragrant.

3. Fluff the cooked brown rice with a fork and transfer to the skillet with the garlic. Stir in the dried thyme, oregano, and chopped parsley. Season with salt and pepper to taste.

4. Cook for 2•3 minutes, stirring frequently, to allow the flavors to meld.

5. Serve the brown rice with herbs warm. Enjoy!

The herbs add great flavor to the nutty brown rice. This makes a simple, healthy side dish. You can adjust the herb amounts to your taste preferences.

66. Grilled Zucchini with Parmesan

Ingredient:

• 3 medium zucchini, sliced lengthwise into 1/4•inch thick slices
• 1 tablespoon olive oil
• 1/4 cup grated Parmesan cheese
• 1 tablespoon chopped fresh basil
• 1/4 teaspoon garlic powder
• Salt and pepper to taste

Instructions:

1. Preheat grill or grill pan to medium•high heat.

2. Brush the zucchini slices lightly with olive oil on both sides.

3. Grill the zucchini slices for 2•3 minutes per side, until tender and lightly charred.

4. Transfer the grilled zucchini to a serving platter.

5. Sprinkle the grated Parmesan cheese, chopped basil, and garlic powder evenly over the top.

6. Season with a pinch of salt and pepper.

7. Serve the grilled zucchini with Parmesan warm.

This recipe follows the DASH diet principles in the following ways:

• Uses heart•healthy olive oil instead of butter or other fats
• Includes vegetables (zucchini) as the main component
• Uses herbs and spices (basil, garlic powder) for flavor instead of relying on salt
• Incorporates a small amount of Parmesan cheese for flavor without going overboard on saturated fat

Additionally, this dish is suitable for renal health as it is low in sodium and potassium. Zucchini is a low•potassium vegetable, making it a good choice for those on a renal diet.

67. Baked Sweet Potato Wedges

Ingredient:

• 3 medium sweet potatoes, scrubbed clean
• 2 tablespoons olive oil
• 1 teaspoon paprika
• 1/2 teaspoon garlic powder
• 1/2 teaspoon dried thyme
• 1/4 teaspoon salt
• 1/4 teaspoon black pepper

Instructions:

1. Preheat the oven to 400°F. Line a large baking sheet with parchment paper.

2. Cut the sweet potatoes in half lengthwise, then cut each half into 4•6 wedges, depending on the size of the potato.

3. Place the sweet potato wedges in a large bowl. Drizzle with the olive oil and toss to coat evenly.

4. In a small bowl, mix together the paprika, garlic powder, dried thyme, salt, and black pepper.

5. Sprinkle the seasoning mixture over the sweet potato wedges and toss to coat evenly.

6. Arrange the seasoned sweet potato wedges in a single layer on the prepared baking sheet.

7. Bake for 25•30 minutes, flipping the wedges halfway through, until tender and lightly browned.

8. Serve the baked sweet potato wedges hot, garnished with any extra seasoning if desired.

These baked sweet potato wedges make a delicious and healthy side dish. The combination of spices adds great flavor. Sweet potatoes are a nutritious vegetable high in vitamins A and C, as well as fiber.

68. Sautéed Spinach with Garlic

Ingredient:

• 1 lb fresh spinach, washed and stems removed
• 1 tablespoon olive oil
• 3 cloves garlic, minced
• 1/4 teaspoon red pepper flakes (optional)
• Salt and pepper to taste

Instructions:

1. In a large skillet or sauté pan, heat the olive oil over medium heat.

2. Add the minced garlic and red pepper flakes (if using) to the pan. Cook for 1 minute, stirring constantly, until fragrant.

3. Add the fresh spinach to the pan in batches, stirring frequently, until the spinach is wilted down, about 3•5 minutes total.

4. Season the sautéed spinach with a pinch of salt and black pepper to taste.

5. Serve the sautéed spinach with garlic warm.

This recipe follows the DASH diet principles in the following ways:

• Uses heart•healthy olive oil instead of butter or other fats
• Includes vegetables (spinach) as the main component
• Uses garlic and red pepper flakes for flavor instead of relying on salt
• Is low in sodium and potassium, making it suitable for a renal diet

Spinach is a nutrient•dense leafy green that is low in potassium, making it a great choice for those on a renal diet. The minimal seasoning allows the fresh flavor of the spinach to shine through.

This simple sautéed spinach dish makes a great side to accompany lean proteins, whole grains, or other DASH•friendly meals.

69. Roasted Carrots with Thyme

Ingredient:

- 1 lb carrots, peeled and cut into 1•inch pieces
- 1 tablespoon olive oil
- 1 teaspoon dried thyme
- 1/4 teaspoon garlic powder
- 1/4 teaspoon salt
- 1/8 teaspoon black pepper

Instructions:

1. Preheat the oven to 400°F. Line a baking sheet with parchment paper.

2. In a large bowl, toss the carrot pieces with the olive oil, dried thyme, garlic powder, salt, and black pepper until evenly coated.

3. Spread the seasoned carrots in a single layer on the prepared baking sheet.

4. Roast the carrots for 20•25 minutes, stirring halfway, until tender and lightly browned.

5. Serve the roasted carrots with thyme warm.

This recipe follows the DASH diet principles in the following ways:

- Uses heart•healthy olive oil instead of butter or other fats
- Includes vegetables (carrots) as the main component
- Uses herbs and spices (thyme, garlic powder) for flavor instead of relying on salt
- Is low in sodium and potassium, making it suitable for a renal diet

Carrots are a great vegetable choice for those on a renal diet, as they are low in potassium. The simple seasoning of thyme, garlic powder, salt, and pepper allows the natural sweetness of the carrots to shine.

This roasted carrot dish makes a delicious and nutritious side to accompany lean proteins or other DASH•friendly meals. It's an easy way to incorporate more vegetables into your diet.

70. Green Beans with Almonds

Ingredient:

• 1 lb fresh green beans, trimmed
• 1 tablespoon olive oil
• 2 tablespoons sliced almonds
• 1 clove garlic, minced
• 1/4 teaspoon dried thyme
• 1/4 teaspoon salt
• 1/8 teaspoon black pepper

Instructions:

1. Bring a large pot of salted water to a boil. Add the trimmed green beans and cook for 5•7 minutes, until tender•crisp. Drain and set aside.

2. In a skillet, heat the olive oil over medium heat. Add the sliced almonds and cook for 2•3 minutes, stirring frequently, until lightly toasted.

3. Add the minced garlic and dried thyme to the skillet. Cook for 1 minute, stirring constantly, until fragrant.

4. Add the cooked green beans to the skillet and toss to coat with the almond mixture. Season with salt and black pepper.

5. Cook for an additional 2•3 minutes, stirring frequently, to allow the flavors to meld. Serve the green beans with almonds warm.

This recipe follows the DASH diet principles in the following ways:

• Uses heart•healthy olive oil instead of butter or other fats
• Includes vegetables (green beans) as the main component
• Uses nuts (almonds) for a source of healthy fats
• Uses herbs and spices (thyme, garlic) for flavor instead of relying on salt
• Is low in sodium and potassium, making it suitable for a renal diet

Green beans are a low•potassium vegetable, making them a great choice for those on a renal diet. The addition of toasted almonds provides a nice crunch and healthy fats to this simple side dish.

This green bean and almond recipe makes a delicious and nutritious accompaniment to lean proteins or other DASH•friendly meals.

71. Fresh Fruit with a Dollop of Greek Yogurt

Ingredient:

• 2 cups mixed fresh fruit (such as berries, sliced peaches, mango, etc.)
• 1 cup plain Greek yogurt
• 1 tablespoon honey (optional)
• 1/4 teaspoon vanilla extract (optional)

Instructions:

1. Wash and prepare the fresh fruit, cutting into bite•sized pieces if necessary.

2. Divide the fresh fruit evenly among 4 serving bowls or plates.

3. Top each serving of fruit with 1/4 cup of plain Greek yogurt.

4. If desired, drizzle a teaspoon of honey over the yogurt and fruit in each bowl.

5. Optionally, add a small dash of vanilla extract to the yogurt.

6. Serve the fresh fruit with a dollop of Greek yogurt immediately.

This recipe follows the DASH diet principles in the following ways:

• Includes fresh fruit as the main component, which is high in fiber, vitamins, and minerals
• Uses plain Greek yogurt, which is a good source of protein and calcium
• Honey is used sparingly as an optional sweetener, rather than relying on added sugars
• The recipe is low in sodium and potassium, making it suitable for a renal diet

Greek yogurt is a great choice for those on a renal diet, as it is lower in potassium compared to regular yogurt. The fresh fruit provides natural sweetness and additional nutrients.

This simple, healthy dessert or snack is a great way to satisfy a sweet craving while following the DASH diet guidelines. It's a refreshing and nutritious option that can be enjoyed any time of day.

72. Baked Apple with Cinnamon

Ingredient:

• 4 medium apples, cored and halved
• 2 tablespoons brown sugar (or maple syrup)
• 1 teaspoon ground cinnamon
• 1/4 cup water

Instructions:

1. Preheat the oven to 375°F. Lightly grease a baking dish or line it with parchment paper.

2. Place the apple halves in the prepared baking dish, cut•side up.

3. In a small bowl, mix together the brown sugar (or maple syrup) and ground cinnamon. Sprinkle the cinnamon•sugar mixture evenly over the apple halves.

4. Pour the water into the bottom of the baking dish, being careful not to pour it directly on the apples.

5. Bake for 25•30 minutes, or until the apples are tender when pierced with a fork.

6. Serve the baked apples warm, spooning any juices from the baking dish over the top.

This recipe follows the DASH diet principles in the following ways:

• Uses a small amount of brown sugar or maple syrup as a natural sweetener, rather than relying on added sugars
• Includes fruit (apples) as the main component
• Uses cinnamon for flavor instead of relying on salt
• Is low in sodium and potassium, making it suitable for a renal diet

Apples are a low•potassium fruit, making them a great choice for those on a renal diet. The baking process brings out the natural sweetness of the apples, while the cinnamon adds warmth and flavor.

This simple baked apple dish can be enjoyed as a healthy dessert or a comforting snack. It's a great way to satisfy a sweet craving while following the DASH diet guidelines.

73. Chia Seed Pudding with Berries

Ingredient:

- 1/4 cup chia seeds
- 1 cup unsweetened almond milk (or low•fat dairy milk)
- 1 tablespoon honey (or maple syrup)
- 1/2 teaspoon vanilla extract
- 1 cup mixed berries (such as raspberries, blueberries, strawberries)

Instructions:

1. In a medium bowl, whisk together the chia seeds, almond milk, honey (or maple syrup), and vanilla extract until well combined.

2. Cover the bowl and refrigerate for at least 2 hours, or up to 24 hours, stirring occasionally, until the chia seeds have thickened the mixture into a pudding•like consistency.

3. When ready to serve, divide the chia seed pudding evenly among 4 serving bowls or glasses.

4. Top each serving with 1/4 cup of the mixed berries.

5. Serve the chia seed pudding with berries chilled.

This recipe follows the DASH diet principles in the following ways:

- Uses unsweetened almond milk or low•fat dairy milk, which are low in sodium and potassium
- Incorporates chia seeds, which are a good source of fiber, protein, and healthy fats
- Includes fresh berries, which are high in antioxidants and low in potassium
- Uses a small amount of honey or maple syrup as a natural sweetener, rather than added sugars

Chia seeds are a great choice for those on a renal diet, as they are low in potassium. The berries provide natural sweetness and additional nutrients without contributing too much potassium.

This chia seed pudding with berries makes a delicious and nutritious breakfast, snack, or dessert that follows the DASH diet principles and is suitable for renal health.

74. Low•Fat Frozen Yogurt

Ingredient:

• 2 cups plain low•fat Greek yogurt
• 1/4 cup honey (or maple syrup)
• 1 teaspoon vanilla extract
• 1/4 teaspoon ground cinnamon (optional)

Instructions:

1. In a medium bowl, whisk together the plain low•fat Greek yogurt, honey (or maple syrup), and vanilla extract until well combined.

2. If desired, stir in the ground cinnamon.

3. Pour the yogurt mixture into an ice cream maker and churn according to the manufacturer's instructions, usually 20•30 minutes.

4. Once the frozen yogurt has reached your desired consistency, transfer it to an airtight container and freeze for at least 2 hours before serving.

5. Scoop and serve the low•fat frozen yogurt in bowls or cones.

This recipe follows the DASH diet principles in the following ways:

• Uses low•fat Greek yogurt as the base, which is a good source of protein and calcium

• Incorporates a small amount of honey or maple syrup as a natural sweetener, rather than added sugars

• The addition of cinnamon provides flavor without relying on salt

• Is low in sodium and potassium, making it suitable for a renal diet

Greek yogurt is a great choice for those on a renal diet, as it is lower in potassium compared to regular yogurt. The frozen yogurt texture provides a refreshing and satisfying treat without the high fat and sugar content of traditional ice cream.

This low•fat frozen yogurt makes a delicious and healthy dessert or snack that aligns with the DASH diet guidelines and is suitable for renal health.

75. Berry Compote with a Touch of Honey

Ingredient:

• 2 cups mixed berries (such as raspberries, blackberries, blueberries)
• 1 tablespoon honey
• 1 tablespoon water
• 1 teaspoon lemon juice
• 1/4 teaspoon ground cinnamon (optional)

Instructions:
1. In a small saucepan, combine the mixed berries, honey, water, and lemon juice.

2. Bring the mixture to a gentle simmer over medium heat, stirring occasionally, until the berries start to break down and release their juices, about 5•7 minutes.

3. If using, stir in the ground cinnamon.

4. Reduce the heat to low and continue to simmer, stirring occasionally, until the compote has thickened slightly, about 5 more minutes.

5. Remove the berry compote from the heat and let it cool slightly.

6. Serve the warm or chilled berry compote over yogurt, oatmeal, or as a topping for other DASH•friendly desserts.

This recipe follows the DASH diet principles in the following ways:
• Uses a variety of low•potassium berries as the main ingredient

• Incorporates a small amount of honey as a natural sweetener, rather than added sugars

• The addition of lemon juice and cinnamon (optional) provides flavor without relying on salt. Is low in sodium and potassium, making it suitable for a renal diet

Berries are an excellent choice for those on a renal diet, as they are low in potassium. The honey adds a touch of sweetness without significantly increasing the sugar content.

This versatile berry compote can be enjoyed as a topping for yogurt, oatmeal, or other DASH•friendly dishes. It's a delicious and nutritious way to incorporate more fruit into your diet while following the DASH diet guidelines and supporting renal health.

76. Poached Pears

Ingredient:

• 4 ripe but firm pears, peeled, halved, and cored
• 2 cups unsweetened apple juice or white wine
• 2 tablespoons honey
• 1 cinnamon stick
• 1 vanilla bean, split lengthwise (or 1 teaspoon vanilla extract)
• 1 strip of lemon zest

Instructions:

1. In a medium saucepan, combine the apple juice (or white wine), honey, cinnamon stick, vanilla bean (or extract), and lemon zest. Bring the mixture to a gentle simmer over medium heat, stirring occasionally until the honey has dissolved.

2. Carefully add the pear halves to the simmering liquid, making sure they are submerged. Reduce the heat to low, cover the pan, and poach the pears for 15•20 minutes, or until they are tender when pierced with a fork.

3. Using a slotted spoon, transfer the poached pear halves to a serving dish.

4. Continue simmering the poaching liquid for 5•10 minutes, or until it has reduced and thickened slightly. Pour the warm poaching liquid over the pears. Serve the poached pears warm or chilled.

This recipe follows the DASH diet principles in the following ways:

• Uses pears, which are a low•potassium fruit, as the main ingredient
• Incorporates a small amount of honey as a natural sweetener, rather than added sugars
• The poaching liquid is flavored with cinnamon, vanilla, and lemon zest, providing flavor without relying on salt
• Is low in sodium and potassium, making it suitable for a renal diet

Pears are an excellent choice for those on a renal diet, as they are low in potassium. The poaching process gently cooks the pears, bringing out their natural sweetness and creating a delicious, healthy dessert.

This poached pear dish can be enjoyed on its own or served with a dollop of low•fat Greek yogurt for an extra protein boost. It's a simple, yet elegant, DASH•friendly dessert that supports renal health.

77. Mango Sorbet

Ingredient:

• 2 cups chopped fresh mango (about 2 medium mangoes)
• 1/4 cup water
• 2 tablespoons honey (or maple syrup)
• 1 tablespoon fresh lime juice

Instructions:

1. In a blender or food processor, combine the chopped mango, water, honey (or maple syrup), and lime juice. Blend until smooth and creamy.

2. Pour the mango mixture into a shallow baking dish or metal pan and place in the freezer.

3. Every 30 minutes, remove the pan from the freezer and stir the mixture with a fork to break up any ice crystals that form. This helps create a smooth, creamy texture.

4. Continue this process for 2•3 hours, or until the sorbet has reached your desired consistency.

5. Once the sorbet is fully frozen, scoop it into serving bowls or cups and serve immediately.

This recipe follows the DASH diet principles in the following ways:

• Uses fresh mango as the main ingredient, which is a low•potassium fruit
• Incorporates a small amount of honey (or maple syrup) as a natural sweetener, rather than added sugars
• The addition of lime juice provides a refreshing, tart flavor without relying on salt
• Is low in sodium and potassium, making it suitable for a renal diet

Mango is an excellent choice for those on a renal diet, as it is low in potassium. The sorbet texture provides a refreshing and satisfying dessert or snack that aligns with the DASH diet guidelines.

This mango sorbet is a delicious and healthy way to enjoy a sweet treat while supporting your renal health. It's a great option for hot summer days or as a palate•cleansing dessert.

78. Dark Chocolate (in moderation)

Ingredient:

• 1 oz high•quality dark chocolate (70% cacao or higher)

Instructions:
1. Savor a small 1 oz serving of dark chocolate. Dark chocolate is rich in antioxidants and can provide health benefits when consumed in moderation.

2. Slowly enjoy the chocolate, allowing it to melt in your mouth. Resist the urge to overindulge, as dark chocolate is still high in calories and fat.

3. Pair the dark chocolate with a cup of herbal tea or a piece of fresh fruit for a satisfying and balanced treat.

Tips:
• Stick to a 1 oz serving size, which is about 1•2 squares of a dark chocolate bar.

• Choose dark chocolate with a high cacao percentage, ideally 70% or higher, for maximum health benefits.

• Savor the chocolate slowly to fully appreciate the rich, complex flavors.

• Enjoy dark chocolate as an occasional treat, not a daily indulgence, to maintain moderation.

Remember, while dark chocolate can be part of a healthy diet, it should be consumed in small portions as part of an overall balanced lifestyle. Moderation is key when it comes to enjoying the benefits of dark chocolate.

79. Grilled Pineapple with a Dash of Cinnamon

Ingredient:

- 1 fresh pineapple, peeled, cored, and cut into 1/2•inch thick slices
- 1 tbsp olive oil or coconut oil
- 1/4 tsp ground cinnamon
- 1 tbsp honey or maple syrup (optional)

Instructions:

1. Preheat your grill or grill pan to medium•high heat.

2. Brush the pineapple slices lightly with the oil on both sides.

3. Sprinkle the cinnamon evenly over the pineapple slices.

4. Grill the pineapple slices for 2•3 minutes per side, until you see grill marks and the fruit is slightly softened.

5. If desired, drizzle the grilled pineapple slices with a small amount of honey or maple syrup just before serving.

6. Serve the warm, grilled pineapple slices immediately, either on their own or paired with grilled meats, yogurt, or ice cream.

The cinnamon adds a warm, spicy note that complements the natural sweetness of the grilled pineapple. This simple, healthy dessert or side dish is perfect for summer cookouts and gatherings.

80. Banana Ice Cream (frozen bananas blended until creamy)

Ingredient:

• 3•4 ripe bananas, peeled and frozen
• 1•2 tbsp unsweetened almond milk or low•fat milk (optional)

Instructions:

1. Peel the ripe bananas and place them in a single layer on a baking sheet or plate. Freeze for at least 2•3 hours, or until completely frozen.

2. Once the bananas are frozen, add them to a high•powered blender or food processor.

3. Blend the frozen bananas, stopping to scrape down the sides as needed, until they reach a smooth, creamy, and ice cream•like consistency. This may take 2•3 minutes of blending.

4. If the mixture seems too thick, add 1•2 tablespoons of unsweetened almond milk or low•fat milk and blend again until desired consistency is reached.

5. Serve the banana ice cream immediately for a soft, creamy texture. For a firmer consistency, transfer the ice cream to an airtight container and freeze for an additional 30 minutes to 1 hour before serving.

Tips:
• Use ripe, spotty bananas for maximum sweetness.

• Avoid adding any additional sweeteners, as the bananas provide natural sweetness.

• This recipe is dairy•free, low in sodium, and suitable for a DASH diet or renal•friendly diet.

• Top with a sprinkle of cinnamon, chopped nuts, or fresh berries for extra flavor and nutrition.

Enjoy this simple, healthy, and delicious banana ice cream as a refreshing treat!

81. Herbal Tea

Ingredient:

• 1•2 teaspoons dried chamomile flowers
• 1 cup (8 oz) hot water

Instructions:
1. Bring the water to a boil.

2. Place the dried chamomile flowers in a tea infuser, tea ball, or directly into a mug.

3. Pour the hot water over the chamomile.

4. Allow the tea to steep for 5•7 minutes.

5. Remove the chamomile flowers or strain the tea.

6. You can add a bit of honey or lemon to taste if desired.

Tips:
• Use 1 teaspoon of chamomile for a lighter tea, or 2 teaspoons for a stronger brew.

• Chamomile tea has a sweet, floral flavor. It's known for its calming and soothing properties.

• You can reuse the chamomile flowers a few times to get multiple cups of tea.

• Drink chamomile tea hot or chilled, depending on your preference.

Enjoy your relaxing cup of chamomile tea!

82. Infused Water with Cucumber and Mint

Ingredient:

- 1 cucumber, sliced
- 1 cup fresh mint leaves
- 8 cups cold water

Instructions:

1. In a large pitcher or beverage dispenser, add the sliced cucumber and mint leaves.

2. Pour the cold water over the cucumber and mint.

3. Stir gently to combine.

4. Refrigerate for at least 2 hours, or up to 8 hours, to allow the flavors to infuse the water.

5. Serve the infused water over ice. You can refill the pitcher with more water as you drink it to continue extracting the flavors.

Tips:
- Use a combination of cucumber and mint, or experiment with other fruit/herb combinations like lemon and rosemary or strawberry and basil.

- For a stronger flavor, muddle the mint leaves slightly before adding to the water.

- Adjust the amount of cucumber and mint to your taste preferences.

- Store the infused water in the refrigerator for up to 3 days.

This refreshing infused water is a great way to stay hydrated and add some natural flavor to your day. Enjoy!

83. Freshly Squeezed Lemonade (low sugar)

Ingredient:

• 6 lemons, juiced (about 1 cup of lemon juice)
• 4 cups cold water
• 2•3 tablespoons honey or maple syrup (to taste)
• Ice cubes

Instructions:

1. In a pitcher, combine the freshly squeezed lemon juice and cold water. Stir to mix.

2. Taste the lemonade and start by adding 2 tablespoons of honey or maple syrup. Stir to dissolve.

3. Adjust the sweetener to your taste preference, adding up to 1 more tablespoon if desired. The amount of sweetener needed will depend on the tartness of your lemons.

4. Fill glasses with ice cubes and pour the lemonade over the top.

5. Serve immediately and enjoy!

Tips:
• Use ripe, juicy lemons for the best flavor.

• Start with less sweetener and add more if needed. The lemonade should have a nice balance of tart and sweet.

• For an extra boost of flavor, add a few lemon slices to the pitcher.

• Store any leftover lemonade in the refrigerator for up to 3 days.

This low•sugar lemonade is a refreshing and healthier alternative to store•bought versions. Adjust the sweetener to your liking for the perfect homemade lemonade!

84. Green Smoothie with Kale and Apple

Ingredient:

- 1 cup packed kale, stems removed
- 1 medium apple, cored and chopped
- 1 cup unsweetened almond milk
- 1/2 cup plain Greek yogurt
- 1 tablespoon honey (optional)
- 1 teaspoon ground cinnamon
- 1/2 teaspoon ground ginger
- Ice cubes (optional)

Instructions:

1. Add the kale, apple, almond milk, Greek yogurt, honey (if using), cinnamon, and ginger to a high•powered blender.

2. Blend on high speed until the mixture is smooth and creamy, about 1•2 minutes.

3. If a thinner consistency is desired, add a few ice cubes and blend again briefly.

4. Pour the smoothie into a glass and enjoy immediately.

Nutritional Benefits:

• Kale is a nutrient•dense leafy green that is low in potassium, making it a great choice for those with kidney concerns.

• Apples provide fiber, vitamin C, and antioxidants without adding too much sugar.

• Greek yogurt adds protein and calcium while keeping the smoothie low in sodium.

• The DASH diet•friendly spices, cinnamon and ginger, provide additional health benefits.

This green smoothie is a great way to start the day or enjoy as a healthy snack. It's packed with vitamins, minerals, and fiber to support overall health and renal function.

85. Berry Smoothie with Almond Milk

Ingredient:

• 1 cup unsweetened almond milk
• 1 cup frozen mixed berries (such as blueberries, raspberries, and blackberries)
• 1/2 banana, frozen
• 1 tablespoon honey (optional)
• 1 tablespoon ground flaxseed (optional)

Instructions:

1. Add the almond milk, frozen berries, and frozen banana to a high•powered blender.

2. Blend on high speed until the mixture is smooth and creamy, about 1•2 minutes.

3. If desired, add the honey and ground flaxseed, and blend again briefly to incorporate.

4. Pour the smoothie into a glass and enjoy immediately.

Tips:
• Use a variety of frozen berries for maximum flavor and nutrition.

• Freeze the banana ahead of time for a thicker, creamier smoothie.

• Adjust the amount of honey to your desired sweetness level.

• The ground flaxseed adds extra fiber and healthy omega•3 fatty acids.

Nutritional Benefits:
• Almond milk is a great dairy•free alternative that is low in calories and high in vitamin E.

• Berries are packed with antioxidants, fiber, and various vitamins and minerals.

• Bananas provide potassium and natural sweetness.

• Honey and flaxseed offer additional health benefits.

This berry smoothie is a refreshing and nutritious way to start your day or enjoy as a healthy snack. The almond milk provides a creamy base while the berries and banana give it a delicious fruity flavor.

86. Iced Green Tea with Lemon

Ingredient:

• 4 green tea bags
• 4 cups water
• 2 tablespoons honey (or to taste)
• 1 lemon, juiced

Instructions:

1. Bring the 4 cups of water to a boil in a saucepan. Remove from heat and add the 4 green tea bags. Let steep for 3•5 minutes.

2. Remove the tea bags and stir in the honey until dissolved.

3. Pour the green tea into a pitcher and refrigerate until completely chilled, about 2 hours.

4. Just before serving, stir in the lemon juice.

5. Fill glasses with ice and pour the iced green tea over the ice. Garnish with lemon slices if desired.

Enjoy your refreshing iced green tea! The lemon adds a nice bright flavor to complement the green tea. Adjust the honey to your desired sweetness level.

87. Low•Sodium Tomato Juice

Ingredient:

• 6 lbs ripe tomatoes, chopped
• 1 cup low•sodium vegetable broth
• 2 tbsp lemon juice
• 1 tsp dried basil
• 1/2 tsp dried oregano
• 1/4 tsp black pepper
• 1/8 tsp salt (optional)

Instructions:

1. In a large pot, combine the chopped tomatoes and vegetable broth. Bring to a boil over medium•high heat.

2. Reduce heat and simmer for 20•25 minutes, stirring occasionally, until tomatoes are very soft.

3. Remove from heat and use an immersion blender to puree the mixture until smooth.

4. Stir in the lemon juice, basil, oregano, and black pepper. Taste and add a small amount of salt if desired, but keep sodium content low.

5. Pour the tomato juice into a pitcher or jars and refrigerate until chilled, at least 2 hours.

This low•sodium tomato juice is perfect for the DASH diet, which emphasizes fruits, vegetables, and low•fat dairy while limiting sodium, saturated fat, and added sugars. It's also a great option for those with kidney disease who need to limit sodium intake. Enjoy this refreshing and healthy beverage!

88. Coconut Water

Ingredient:

- 1 cup coconut water
- 1/4 cup chia seeds
- 2 tbsp maple syrup or honey (or your preferred sweetener)
- 1/2 tsp vanilla extract
- Pinch of salt
- Toppings (such as fresh fruit, toasted coconut, nuts, etc.)

Instructions:

1. In a medium bowl, whisk together the coconut water, chia seeds, maple syrup/honey, vanilla, and salt until well combined.

2. Cover the bowl and refrigerate for at least 2 hours, or up to overnight, stirring occasionally, until the chia seeds have thickened the mixture into a pudding•like consistency.

3. Divide the chia pudding into serving bowls or jars. Top with your desired toppings such as fresh fruit, toasted coconut, nuts, etc.

4. Serve chilled. The chia pudding will keep refrigerated for up to 5 days.

Variations:
- Use different fruit purees or juices instead of coconut water.

- Add a spoonful of peanut butter or almond butter.

- Sprinkle with cinnamon or cocoa powder.

- Use different sweeteners like agave, date syrup, or stevia.

Enjoy this healthy, hydrating, and delicious coconut water chia pudding!

89. Carrot and Orange Juice

Ingredient:

- 6 medium carrots, peeled and chopped
- 3 oranges, peeled and segmented
- 1/2 cup water (optional)
- 1 tbsp fresh lemon juice (optional)

Instructions:

1. In a juicer, juice the carrots and orange segments together until you have about 12 ounces of juice.

2. If the juice is too thick, add the 1/2 cup of water and stir to thin it out.

3. Stir in the lemon juice, if using, to add a touch of acidity and balance the sweetness.

4. Pour the carrot and orange juice into glasses and serve immediately.

This juice is a great option for the DASH diet, which emphasizes fruits and vegetables. Carrots are a good source of vitamins, minerals, and antioxidants, while oranges provide vitamin C and other beneficial compounds.

For those following a renal diet, this juice is relatively low in potassium and phosphorus, making it a suitable choice. Just be mindful of portion sizes, as even healthy juices can be high in natural sugars.

Enjoy this refreshing and nutritious carrot and orange juice! It's a great way to start the day or have as a healthy snack.

90. Hibiscus Tea

Ingredient:

- 4 cups water
- 1/2 cup dried hibiscus flowers (or 4•5 hibiscus tea bags)
- 2•3 tbsp honey or agave nectar (optional)
- 1 tbsp fresh lemon juice (optional)

Instructions:

1. In a medium saucepan, bring the 4 cups of water to a boil.

2. Remove the pan from heat and add the dried hibiscus flowers (or tea bags). Cover and let steep for 5•7 minutes.

3. Strain the tea through a fine•mesh sieve to remove the hibiscus flowers. Discard the flowers.

4. Stir in the honey or agave nectar, if using, until dissolved. Start with 2 tbsp and add more to taste if desired.

5. Stir in the lemon juice, if using, to add a touch of acidity and balance the sweetness.

6. Pour the hibiscus tea into glasses and serve hot or chilled over ice.

Hibiscus tea is a great option for the DASH diet, as it is naturally low in calories, sodium, and sugar. It's also a good source of vitamin C and antioxidants.

For those following a renal diet, hibiscus tea is generally considered safe and low in potassium and phosphorus. However, as with any beverage, it's important to monitor portion sizes and fluid intake.

Enjoy this refreshing and vibrant hibiscus tea! It's a delicious and healthy alternative to sugary drinks.

91. Whole Wheat Pita with Hummus and Veggies

Ingredient:

- 2 whole wheat pita breads, halved
- 1/2 cup hummus (store•bought or homemade)
- 1 cup sliced cucumber
- 1 cup sliced bell pepper (any color)
- 1/2 cup cherry tomatoes, halved
- 2 tbsp crumbled feta cheese (optional)
- 1 tbsp chopped fresh parsley (optional)

Instructions:

1. Toast the whole wheat pita halves until lightly crisp.

2. Spread about 2 tablespoons of hummus onto each pita half.

3. Top the hummus with the sliced cucumber, bell pepper, and cherry tomatoes.

4. Sprinkle the crumbled feta cheese and chopped parsley over the top, if using.

5. Serve the whole wheat pita with hummus and veggies immediately.

This snack or light meal is a great option for the DASH diet, as it is high in fiber, vitamins, and minerals from the whole grains, vegetables, and hummus. The hummus provides plant•based protein, while the feta cheese (if used) adds a small amount of dairy.

For those following a renal diet, this recipe is relatively low in sodium, potassium, and phosphorus, making it a suitable choice. Just be mindful of portion sizes, as pita bread and hummus can be higher in carbohydrates.

Enjoy this delicious and nutritious whole wheat pita with hummus and fresh veggies!

92. Baked Cod with Lemon and Dill

Ingredient:

• 1 lb cod fillets, cut into 4 portions
• 2 tablespoons fresh lemon juice
• 1 tablespoon chopped fresh dill
• 1 teaspoon grated lemon zest
• 1/4 teaspoon black pepper
• Cooking spray

Instructions:

1. Preheat the oven to 400°F. Lightly coat a baking dish with cooking spray.

2. Place the cod fillets in the prepared baking dish. Drizzle the lemon juice over the top.

3. In a small bowl, mix together the dill, lemon zest, and black pepper. Sprinkle the mixture evenly over the cod.

4. Bake for 12•15 minutes, or until the cod flakes easily with a fork and is opaque throughout.

5. Serve the baked cod immediately, garnished with additional fresh dill if desired.

Nutritional Benefits:
• Cod is a lean, low•sodium fish that is an excellent source of protein.
• Lemon and dill provide bright, fresh flavors without adding any sodium.
• This recipe is low in calories, fat, and sodium, making it suitable for the DASH diet and renal•friendly diets.

Tips:
• Use fresh, high•quality cod for the best texture and flavor.
• Adjust the baking time based on the thickness of your cod fillets.
• Serve the baked cod with roasted vegetables or a side salad for a complete, healthy meal.

This Baked Cod with Lemon and Dill is a simple, delicious, and nutritious dish that fits well within the DASH diet guidelines and is kidney•friendly.

93. Grilled Chicken Salad with Avocado

Ingredient:

• 4 boneless, skinless chicken breasts
• 1 tbsp olive oil
• 1 tsp dried oregano
• 1/4 tsp black pepper
• 1/8 tsp salt (optional)
• 8 cups mixed greens
 (such as spinach, romaine, and arugula)
• 1 avocado, sliced
• 1 cup cherry tomatoes, halved
• 1/4 cup sliced cucumber
• 2 tbsp crumbled feta cheese (optional)
• 2 tbsp balsamic vinaigrette (recipe below)

Balsamic Vinaigrette:
• 2 tbsp balsamic vinegar
• 1 tbsp olive oil
• 1 tsp Dijon mustard
• 1 tsp honey
• 1/4 tsp black pepper

Instructions:

1. Preheat grill or grill pan to medium·high heat.

2. Rub the chicken breasts with the olive oil, oregano, black pepper, and a small amount of salt (if using).

3. Grill the chicken for 6·8 minutes per side, or until cooked through. Let rest for 5 minutes, then slice or chop the chicken.

4. In a large salad bowl, combine the mixed greens, avocado slices, cherry tomatoes, and cucumber.

5. In a small bowl, whisk together the balsamic vinaigrette ingredients.

6. Add the grilled chicken and feta cheese (if using) to the salad. Drizzle the balsamic vinaigrette over the top and toss gently to coat. Serve the grilled chicken salad immediately.

This salad is a great option for the DASH diet, as it is high in vegetables, lean protein, and healthy fats from the avocado, while keeping sodium content low. It's also a suitable choice for those with kidney disease who need to monitor their sodium intake.

94. Turkey and Spinach Wrap

Ingredient:

• 2 whole wheat tortillas or wraps
• 4 oz sliced turkey breast
• 1 cup fresh spinach leaves
• 1/2 avocado, sliced
• 2 tbsp hummus
• 1 tbsp crumbled feta cheese (optional)
• 1 tbsp chopped fresh parsley (optional)
• 1 tsp olive oil
• 1 tsp lemon juice

Instructions:

1. Lay the whole wheat tortillas or wraps on a flat surface.

2. Spread 1 tbsp of hummus evenly over each tortilla.

3. Layer the sliced turkey, spinach leaves, avocado slices, feta cheese (if using), and parsley (if using) onto the tortillas.

4. Drizzle the olive oil and lemon juice over the fillings.

5. Carefully roll up the tortillas tightly, tucking in the sides as you go.

6. Cut the wraps in half diagonally and serve immediately.

This turkey and spinach wrap is a great option for the DASH diet, as it is high in lean protein, vegetables, and healthy fats from the avocado. The whole wheat tortilla provides fiber, and the hummus adds plant·based protein.

For those following a renal diet, this wrap is relatively low in sodium, potassium, and phosphorus, making it a suitable choice. Just be mindful of portion sizes, as the tortilla and hummus can be higher in carbohydrates.

Enjoy this delicious and nutritious turkey and spinach wrap!

95. Veggie Burger on Whole Grain Bun

Ingredient:

- 2 whole grain hamburger buns
- 2 veggie burger patties (store•bought or homemade)
- 1 cup shredded lettuce
- 1/2 tomato, sliced
- 1/4 cup sliced cucumber
- 2 tbsp avocado, mashed
- 1 tbsp low•sodium mustard
- 1 tsp olive oil

Instructions:

1. Toast the whole grain hamburger buns until lightly golden.

2. Cook the veggie burger patties according to package instructions or your homemade recipe.

3. Place the cooked veggie burger patties on the bottom buns.

4. Top the patties with the shredded lettuce, tomato slices, and cucumber slices.

5. Spread the mashed avocado on the top buns.

6. Drizzle the olive oil and spread the low•sodium mustard over the avocado.

7. Close the burgers and serve immediately.

This veggie burger on a whole grain bun is a great option for the DASH diet, as it is high in fiber, vegetables, and plant•based protein from the veggie patty. The whole grain bun provides complex carbohydrates, and the avocado adds healthy fats.

For those following a renal diet, this burger is relatively low in sodium, potassium, and phosphorus, making it a suitable choice. Just be mindful of portion sizes, as the bun and veggie patty can be higher in carbohydrates.

Enjoy this delicious and nutritious veggie burger on a whole grain bun!

96. Tofu and Vegetable Skewers

Ingredient:

- 1 block (14 oz) extra•firm tofu, cut into 1•inch cubes
- 1 red bell pepper, cut into 1•inch pieces
- 1 zucchini, cut into 1/2•inch thick rounds
- 1 red onion, cut into 1•inch pieces
- 8•10 cherry tomatoes
- 2 tbsp olive oil
- 1 tbsp lemon juice
- 1 tsp dried oregano
- 1/4 tsp black pepper
- 1/8 tsp salt (optional)

Instructions:

1. Preheat grill or grill pan to medium•high heat.

2. In a large bowl, gently toss the tofu, bell pepper, zucchini, onion, and cherry tomatoes with the olive oil, lemon juice, oregano, and black pepper. Season with a small amount of salt if desired, but keep sodium content low.

3. Thread the marinated vegetables and tofu onto skewers, alternating the ingredients.

4. Grill the skewers for 10•12 minutes, turning occasionally, until the vegetables are tender and the tofu is lightly charred.

5. Serve the grilled tofu and vegetable skewers immediately.

These skewers are a great option for the DASH diet, which emphasizes plant•based proteins, fruits, and vegetables while limiting sodium, saturated fat, and added sugars. They are also suitable for those with kidney disease who need to monitor their sodium intake. Enjoy this flavorful and healthy grilled dish!

97. Fish Tacos with Cabbage Slaw

Ingredient:

- 1 lb white fish fillets (such as tilapia or cod), cut into 1•inch pieces
- 1 tbsp olive oil
- 1 tsp chili powder
- 1/2 tsp cumin
- 1/4 tsp garlic powder
- 1/4 tsp salt
- 8 small whole wheat tortillas
- 2 cups shredded green cabbage
- 1 cup shredded red cabbage
- 1/4 cup chopped cilantro
- 2 tbsp lime juice
- 1 tbsp olive oil
- 1/4 tsp black pepper
- 2 tbsp low•fat plain Greek yogurt (optional)

Instructions:

1. In a bowl, toss the fish pieces with the 1 tbsp olive oil, chili powder, cumin, garlic powder, and salt.

2. In a separate bowl, combine the shredded green and red cabbage, cilantro, lime juice, 1 tbsp olive oil, and black pepper. Toss to coat.

3. Heat a large skillet or grill pan over medium•high heat. Cook the seasoned fish pieces for 3•4 minutes per side, until opaque and flaky.

4. Warm the whole wheat tortillas according to package instructions.

5. To assemble the tacos, place some of the cooked fish in the center of each tortilla. Top with the cabbage slaw and a dollop of Greek yogurt (if using). Serve the fish tacos immediately.

These fish tacos with cabbage slaw are a great option for the DASH diet, as they are high in lean protein, fiber, and vegetables. The whole wheat tortillas provide complex carbohydrates, while the Greek yogurt (if used) adds a touch of dairy.

For those following a renal diet, this dish is relatively low in sodium, potassium, and phosphorus, making it a suitable choice. Just be mindful of portion sizes, as the tortillas can be higher in carbohydrates.

98. Spaghetti with Lentil Bolognese

Ingredient:

- 8 oz whole wheat spaghetti
- 1 tbsp olive oil
- 1 onion, diced
- 3 garlic cloves, minced
- 1 carrot, peeled and diced
- 1 celery stalk, diced
- 1 cup brown or green lentils, rinsed
- 1 (28 oz) can diced tomatoes
- 2 tbsp tomato paste
- 1 tsp dried oregano
- 1/2 tsp dried basil
- 1/4 tsp black pepper
- 1/8 tsp salt (optional)
- 2 tbsp grated Parmesan cheese (optional)
- Chopped fresh parsley for garnish

Instructions:

1. Cook the whole wheat spaghetti according to package instructions. Drain and set aside.

2. In a large skillet, heat the olive oil over medium heat. Add the onion, garlic, carrot, and celery. Sauté for 5•7 minutes until the vegetables are softened.

3. Add the lentils, diced tomatoes, tomato paste, oregano, basil, black pepper, and a small amount of salt (if using). Stir to combine.

4. Reduce heat to low and simmer the lentil bolognese for 20•25 minutes, stirring occasionally, until the lentils are tender.

5. Serve the lentil bolognese over the cooked whole wheat spaghetti. Top with grated Parmesan cheese (if using) and chopped fresh parsley.

This spaghetti with lentil bolognese is a great option for the DASH diet, as it is high in fiber, plant•based protein, and vegetables. The whole wheat spaghetti provides complex carbohydrates, while the lentils and Parmesan cheese (if used) add a source of protein.

For those following a renal diet, this dish is relatively low in sodium, potassium, and phosphorus, making it a suitable choice. Just be mindful of portion sizes, as pasta can be higher in carbohydrates.

99. Veggie and Hummus Wrap

Ingredient:

• 2 whole wheat tortillas or wraps
• 1/2 cup hummus (store•bought or homemade)
• 1 cup mixed greens (such as spinach, arugula, or kale)
• 1/2 cup sliced cucumber
• 1/2 cup sliced bell pepper
• 1/4 cup shredded carrots
• 2 tbsp crumbled feta cheese (optional)
• 1 tbsp chopped fresh parsley (optional)
• 1 tsp olive oil
• 1 tsp lemon juice

Instructions:

1. Lay the whole wheat tortillas or wraps on a flat surface.

2. Spread 1/4 cup of hummus evenly over each tortilla.

3. Layer the mixed greens, sliced cucumber, bell pepper, and shredded carrots onto the hummus.

4. Sprinkle the crumbled feta cheese and chopped parsley over the vegetables, if using.

5. Drizzle the olive oil and lemon juice over the fillings.

6. Carefully roll up the tortillas tightly, tucking in the sides as you go.

7. Cut the wraps in half diagonally and serve immediately.

This veggie and hummus wrap is a great option for the DASH diet, as it is high in fiber, vitamins, and minerals from the vegetables, while the hummus provides plant•based protein and healthy fats.

For those following a renal diet, this wrap is relatively low in sodium, potassium, and phosphorus, making it a suitable choice. The feta cheese can be omitted or reduced to further lower the sodium content.

Enjoy this delicious and nutritious veggie and hummus wrap as a quick and easy meal or snack that follows the DASH diet principles and is suitable for renal health.

100. Chicken and Quinoa Stuffed Peppers

Ingredient:

• 4 bell peppers (any color), halved and seeded
• 1 cup cooked quinoa
• 1 cup cooked and shredded chicken breast
• 1/2 cup diced tomatoes
• 1/4 cup chopped fresh parsley
• 1 tbsp olive oil
• 1 tsp dried oregano
• 1/4 tsp black pepper
• 1/8 tsp salt (optional)
• 2 tbsp crumbled feta cheese (optional)

Instructions:

1. Preheat the oven to 375°F.

2. Slice the bell peppers in half lengthwise and remove the seeds and membranes.

3. In a medium bowl, combine the cooked quinoa, shredded chicken, diced tomatoes, parsley, olive oil, oregano, black pepper, and a small amount of salt (if using).

4. Stuff the pepper halves evenly with the chicken and quinoa mixture.

5. Place the stuffed pepper halves in a baking dish. Cover with foil.

6. Bake for 25•30 minutes, or until the peppers are tender.

7. Remove the foil and sprinkle the crumbled feta cheese (if using) over the top.

8. Serve the chicken and quinoa stuffed peppers warm.

This dish is a great option for the DASH diet, as it is high in vegetables, lean protein, and whole grains. The quinoa provides complex carbohydrates and fiber, while the chicken adds protein.

For those following a renal diet, this recipe is relatively low in sodium, potassium, and phosphorus, making it a suitable choice. The optional feta cheese can be omitted or reduced to further lower the sodium content.

101. Whole Grain Rice Cakes with Avocado

Ingredient:

• 2 whole grain rice cakes
• 1/2 ripe avocado, mashed
• 1 tbsp lemon juice
• 1/4 tsp garlic powder
• 1/8 tsp black pepper
• 1/8 tsp salt (optional)

Instructions:

1. In a small bowl, mash the avocado with a fork. Stir in the lemon juice, garlic powder, black pepper, and a small amount of salt (if using).

2. Spread the mashed avocado mixture evenly over the two whole grain rice cakes.

3. Serve the rice cakes with avocado immediately.

This snack of whole grain rice cakes with avocado is a great option for the DASH diet. The whole grain rice cakes provide complex carbohydrates and fiber, while the avocado adds healthy monounsaturated fats, vitamins, and minerals.

For those following a renal diet, this snack is relatively low in sodium, potassium, and phosphorus, making it a suitable choice. The small amount of salt is optional, and can be omitted if needed.

Enjoy this simple yet satisfying snack that combines the creamy texture of avocado with the crunch of whole grain rice cakes. It's a nutritious and DASH•friendly option that can be easily incorporated into your meal plan.

102. Sliced Apples with a Dash of Cinnamon

Ingredient:

• 2 medium apples, cored and sliced
• 1/4 tsp ground cinnamon

Instructions:

1. Wash the apples, core them, and slice them into thin wedges or rounds.

2. Arrange the apple slices on a plate or platter.

3. Sprinkle the ground cinnamon evenly over the apple slices.

That's it! This simple snack is a great option for the DASH diet and those following a renal diet.

Apples are a good source of fiber, vitamins, and antioxidants. The cinnamon adds a warm, sweet flavor without any added sugars or sodium.

This snack is suitable for a renal diet as apples and cinnamon are both low in sodium, potassium, and phosphorus. It's a great way to satisfy a sweet craving while keeping your nutrient intake in check.

Enjoy these sliced apples with a dash of cinnamon as a healthy, DASH•friendly snack or dessert. It's a simple, delicious, and nutritious option that can be easily incorporated into your meal plan.

103. Mixed Nuts and Dried Fruit (unsalted)

Ingredient:

• 1/4 cup raw, unsalted almonds
• 1/4 cup raw, unsalted walnuts
• 1/4 cup raw, unsalted cashews
• 2 tbsp unsweetened dried cranberries
• 2 tbsp unsweetened dried apricots, chopped

Instructions:

1. In a small bowl, combine the raw, unsalted almonds, walnuts, and cashews.

2. Add the unsweetened dried cranberries and chopped dried apricots to the nut mixture.

3. Stir gently to mix the nuts and dried fruit together.

4. Portion the mixed nuts and dried fruit into small containers or snack bags for easy, on•the•go access.

This mixed nuts and dried fruit snack is a great option for the DASH diet, as it provides a balance of healthy fats, fiber, and natural sweetness without added sugars or sodium.

The nuts are a good source of unsaturated fats, protein, and various vitamins and minerals. The dried fruit adds carbohydrates and antioxidants, while keeping the sodium content low.

For those following a renal diet, this snack is relatively low in sodium, potassium, and phosphorus, making it a suitable choice. Just be mindful of portion sizes, as nuts and dried fruit can be high in calories.

Enjoy this nutritious and satisfying mixed nuts and dried fruit snack as part of a DASH•friendly diet or renal•friendly meal plan.

104. Sliced Bell Peppers with Low•Fat Dip

Ingredient:

• 2 bell peppers (any color), sliced into strips
• 1 cup low•fat plain Greek yogurt
• 2 tbsp chopped fresh herbs (such as dill, parsley, or chives)
• 1 tsp lemon juice
• 1/4 tsp garlic powder
• 1/8 tsp salt (optional)
• 1/8 tsp black pepper

Instructions:

1. Wash the bell peppers and slice them into long, thin strips.

2. In a small bowl, combine the low•fat plain Greek yogurt, chopped fresh herbs, lemon juice, garlic powder, and a small amount of salt (if using) and black pepper. Stir to mix well.

3. Arrange the sliced bell pepper strips on a serving platter or plate.

4. Serve the low•fat dip alongside the bell pepper strips for dipping.

This snack of sliced bell peppers with a low•fat dip is a great option for the DASH diet. The bell peppers provide a crunchy, nutrient•dense vegetable, while the low•fat yogurt•based dip adds a creamy, flavorful element.

For those following a renal diet, this dish is relatively low in sodium, potassium, and phosphorus, making it a suitable choice. The Greek yogurt provides a source of protein without being too high in these nutrients.

Enjoy this refreshing and healthy snack! The bell peppers and low•fat dip make for a delicious and satisfying combination.

105. Low•Sodium Cheese and Apple Slices

Ingredient:

• 1 medium apple, cored and sliced
• 1 oz low•sodium cheddar or Swiss cheese, sliced or cubed
• 1 tsp lemon juice (optional)

Instructions:

1. Wash and core the apple, then slice it into thin wedges or slices.

2. Arrange the apple slices on a plate or platter.

3. Place the slices or cubes of low•sodium cheese next to the apple slices.

4. If desired, drizzle the apple slices with a small amount of lemon juice to prevent browning.

That's it! This simple snack or light meal is a great option for the DASH diet and those following a renal diet.

The apple provides fiber, vitamins, and natural sweetness, while the low•sodium cheese adds a source of protein and calcium. The lemon juice is optional, but can help preserve the color of the apple slices.

This combination of crisp apple and creamy, low•sodium cheese is a tasty and nutritious choice. It's perfect for a quick snack or as part of a larger DASH•friendly meal.

Remember to choose low•sodium cheese varieties to keep the sodium content in check, especially for those with kidney concerns. Enjoy this simple but satisfying snack!

106. Hard•Boiled Eggs

Ingredient:

• 6 large eggs

Instructions:

1. Place the eggs in a single layer in a saucepan and cover with cold water by 1 inch.

2. Bring the water to a boil over high heat.

3. Once the water reaches a full boil, remove the pan from the heat and cover with a lid.

4. Let the eggs sit in the hot water for 12 minutes for hard•boiled eggs.

5. Drain the hot water and cover the eggs with cold water to stop the cooking process.

6. Let the eggs sit in the cold water for 5 minutes.

7. Peel the eggs and enjoy as a snack or use in other recipes.

Hard•boiled eggs are a great option for the DASH diet and those following a renal diet. They are a good source of high•quality protein, and they are low in sodium, potassium, and phosphorus.

The DASH diet emphasizes lean proteins, and hard•boiled eggs fit that criteria perfectly. They can be enjoyed on their own as a snack or incorporated into other DASH•friendly dishes, such as salads or sandwiches.

For those with kidney concerns, hard•boiled eggs are a suitable choice, as they are low in the nutrients that may need to be limited on a renal diet. Just be mindful of portion sizes, as eggs can still contribute to overall calorie and cholesterol intake.

Enjoy these simple, nutritious hard•boiled eggs as part of a DASH•friendly and renal•friendly meal plan.

107. Cucumber Slices with Cottage Cheese

Ingredient:

• 1 medium cucumber, sliced into rounds
• 1/2 cup low•fat or non•fat cottage cheese
• 1 tbsp chopped fresh dill (or other fresh herbs)
• 1/4 tsp black pepper

Instructions:

1. Wash the cucumber and slice it into thin, round slices.

2. In a small bowl, mix together the cottage cheese, chopped fresh dill, and black pepper.

3. Arrange the cucumber slices on a plate or platter.

4. Spoon a small amount of the cottage cheese mixture onto each cucumber slice.

That's it! This simple snack or appetizer is a great option for the DASH diet and those following a renal diet.

The cucumber provides hydration, fiber, and vitamins, while the cottage cheese adds protein and calcium. The fresh dill and black pepper add flavor without the need for salt.

This combination of crunchy cucumber and creamy, protein•rich cottage cheese is a tasty and nutritious choice. It's perfect for a quick snack or as part of a larger DASH•friendly meal.

Remember to choose low•fat or non•fat cottage cheese to keep the saturated fat and sodium content low, especially for those with kidney concerns. Enjoy this refreshing and healthy snack!

108. Veggie Chips (baked)

Ingredient:

• 2 medium zucchini, sliced into 1/8•inch thick rounds
• 2 medium carrots, peeled and sliced into 1/8•inch thick rounds
• 1 medium beet, peeled and sliced into 1/8•inch thick rounds
• 1 tbsp olive oil
• 1/2 tsp garlic powder
• 1/4 tsp black pepper
• 1/8 tsp salt (optional)

Instructions:
1. Preheat the oven to 375°F. Line two baking sheets with parchment paper.

2. In a large bowl, toss the sliced zucchini, carrots, and beet rounds with the olive oil, garlic powder, black pepper, and a small amount of salt (if using).

3. Arrange the vegetable slices in a single layer on the prepared baking sheets, making sure they are not overlapping.

4. Bake for 18•22 minutes, flipping the slices halfway through, until the edges are crispy and the centers are tender.

5. Remove the baked veggie chips from the oven and let cool completely before serving.

These baked veggie chips are a great option for the DASH diet and those following a renal diet. They provide a crunchy, flavorful snack that is low in sodium, potassium, and phosphorus.

The variety of vegetables used • zucchini, carrots, and beets • adds a range of vitamins, minerals, and antioxidants. The olive oil and spices provide taste without the need for excessive sodium.

Enjoy these homemade, baked veggie chips as a healthy alternative to traditional potato chips. They make a great snack or side dish that aligns with the DASH diet principles and is suitable for renal health.

109. Homemade Trail Mix

Ingredient:

• 1/2 cup raw, unsalted almonds
• 1/2 cup raw, unsalted walnuts
• 1/4 cup raw, unsalted pumpkin seeds
• 1/4 cup raw, unsalted sunflower seeds
• 2 tbsp unsweetened dried cranberries
• 2 tbsp unsweetened dried apricots, chopped

Instructions:

1. In a medium bowl, combine the raw, unsalted almonds, walnuts, pumpkin seeds, and sunflower seeds.

2. Add the unsweetened dried cranberries and chopped dried apricots to the nut and seed mixture.

3. Stir gently to mix all the ingredients together.

4. Transfer the homemade trail mix to an airtight container or individual snack bags for easy portioning.

This homemade trail mix is a great option for the DASH diet and those following a renal diet. It provides a balance of healthy fats, protein, fiber, and natural sweetness without added sugars or sodium.

The nuts and seeds are a good source of unsaturated fats, protein, and various vitamins and minerals. The dried fruit adds carbohydrates and antioxidants, while keeping the sodium content low.

For those with kidney concerns, this trail mix is relatively low in sodium, potassium, and phosphorus, making it a suitable choice. Just be mindful of portion sizes, as nuts and dried fruit can be high in calories.

Enjoy this nutritious and satisfying homemade trail mix as a snack or addition to your DASH•friendly and renal•friendly meals.

110. Protein Smoothie with Berries and Spinach

Ingredient:

- 1 cup unsweetened almond milk
- 1/2 cup frozen mixed berries (such as blueberries, raspberries, and blackberries)
- 1 cup fresh spinach leaves
- 1/2 banana, frozen
- 2 tbsp unsweetened protein powder (such as whey or plant•based)
- 1 tbsp ground flaxseed (optional)
- 1 tsp honey (optional)

Instructions:

1. In a high•speed blender, combine the unsweetened almond milk, frozen mixed berries, fresh spinach leaves, frozen banana, protein powder, and ground flaxseed (if using).

2. Blend the ingredients on high speed until the smoothie is smooth and creamy, about 1•2 minutes.

3. Taste the smoothie and add a teaspoon of honey if you'd like it to be slightly sweeter.

4. Pour the protein smoothie into a glass and enjoy immediately.

This protein•packed smoothie is a great option for the DASH diet and those following a renal diet. It's high in fiber, vitamins, and minerals from the berries and spinach, while the protein powder and flaxseed provide a boost of protein and healthy fats.

The unsweetened almond milk and optional honey keep the added sugar and sodium content low, making this smoothie a suitable choice for those with kidney concerns.

Enjoy this nutritious and delicious protein smoothie as a quick breakfast, snack, or post•workout recovery drink that aligns with the DASH diet principles and renal health guidelines.

111. Berry Parfait with Low•Fat Yogurt

Ingredient:

- 1 cup low•fat or non•fat plain Greek yogurt
- 1 cup fresh or frozen mixed berries (such as blueberries, raspberries, and blackberries)
- 2 tbsp chopped walnuts (optional)
- 1 tsp honey (optional)

Instructions:

1. In a parfait glass or small bowl, layer half of the yogurt on the bottom.

2. Top the yogurt with half of the mixed berries.

3. Repeat the layers, ending with the berries on top.

4. If desired, sprinkle the chopped walnuts over the top of the parfait.

5. Drizzle the honey over the parfait, if using.

This berry parfait with low•fat yogurt is a great option for the DASH diet and those following a renal diet.

The low•fat or non•fat Greek yogurt provides protein and calcium, while the mixed berries are a source of fiber, vitamins, and antioxidants. The optional walnuts add a crunchy texture and healthy fats.

For those with kidney concerns, this parfait is relatively low in sodium, potassium, and phosphorus. The honey is optional and can be omitted if needed to further reduce the added sugar content.

Enjoy this refreshing and nutritious berry parfait as a healthy breakfast, snack, or dessert that aligns with the DASH diet principles and supports renal health.

112. Whole Wheat Pancakes with Fresh Fruit

Ingredient:

- 1 cup whole wheat flour
- 1 tsp baking powder
- 1/4 tsp baking soda
- 1/4 tsp ground cinnamon
- 1 egg
- 1 cup low•fat or unsweetened almond milk
- 1 tbsp honey (optional)
- 1 cup mixed fresh berries (such as blueberries, raspberries, and sliced strawberries)

Instructions:

1. In a medium bowl, whisk together the whole wheat flour, baking powder, baking soda, and cinnamon.

2. In a separate bowl, beat the egg. Then stir in the low•fat or almond milk and honey (if using).

3. Pour the wet ingredients into the dry ingredients and stir just until combined (do not overmix).

4. Heat a non•stick skillet or griddle over medium heat. Lightly coat with a small amount of oil or non•stick cooking spray.

5. For each pancake, pour about 1/4 cup of the batter onto the hot surface. Cook for 2•3 minutes per side, or until golden brown.

6. Serve the whole wheat pancakes warm, topped with the fresh mixed berries.

These whole wheat pancakes with fresh fruit are a great option for the DASH diet and those following a renal diet. The whole grains, low•fat dairy, and fresh produce provide a nutritious and balanced meal.

The whole wheat flour adds fiber, while the berries are a source of vitamins, minerals, and antioxidants. The optional honey can provide a touch of sweetness without excessive added sugar.

For those with kidney concerns, this recipe is relatively low in sodium, potassium, and phosphorus, making it a suitable choice. Adjust the portion sizes as needed to fit your dietary needs

113. Avocado and Tomato on Whole Grain Toast

Ingredient:

• 2 slices whole grain bread
• 1/2 ripe avocado, mashed
• 1 medium tomato, sliced
• 1 tbsp lemon juice
• 1/4 tsp garlic powder
• 1/8 tsp black pepper
• 1/8 tsp salt (optional)

Instructions:

1. Toast the two slices of whole grain bread until lightly golden.

2. In a small bowl, mash the avocado with a fork. Stir in the lemon juice, garlic powder, black pepper, and a small amount of salt (if using).

3. Spread the mashed avocado mixture evenly over the toasted whole grain bread slices.

4. Top the avocado with the sliced tomatoes.

5. Serve the avocado and tomato on whole grain toast immediately.

This open•faced sandwich is a great option for the DASH diet and those following a renal diet. The whole grain bread provides complex carbohydrates and fiber, while the avocado and tomato offer healthy fats, vitamins, and minerals.

The lemon juice, garlic powder, and small amount of salt (if used) add flavor without the need for excessive sodium. This makes it a suitable choice for those with kidney concerns who need to limit their sodium intake.

Enjoy this nutritious and delicious avocado and tomato on whole grain toast as a quick and easy breakfast, lunch, or snack that aligns with the DASH diet principles and supports renal health.

114. Chia Seed Pudding with Almond Milk

Ingredient:

- 1/4 cup chia seeds
- 1 cup unsweetened almond milk
- 1 tbsp honey (optional)
- 1/2 tsp vanilla extract
- 1/4 tsp ground cinnamon
- 1/4 cup fresh berries (such as blueberries or raspberries)

Instructions:

1. In a medium bowl, whisk together the chia seeds, unsweetened almond milk, honey (if using), vanilla extract, and ground cinnamon until well combined.

2. Cover the bowl and refrigerate the chia seed pudding for at least 2 hours, or overnight, stirring occasionally, until thickened.

3. When ready to serve, spoon the chia seed pudding into individual bowls or glasses.

4. Top each serving with 2•3 tablespoons of fresh berries.

This chia seed pudding with almond milk is a great option for the DASH diet and those following a renal diet.

Chia seeds are a good source of fiber, protein, and omega•3 fatty acids. The unsweetened almond milk provides a dairy•free, low•sodium, and low•potassium base for the pudding. The optional honey adds a touch of sweetness, while the cinnamon provides flavor without the need for salt.

The fresh berries on top add antioxidants, vitamins, and a pop of color and flavor to the pudding.

This recipe is suitable for those with kidney concerns, as it is relatively low in sodium, potassium, and phosphorus. Adjust the portion sizes as needed to fit your dietary requirements.

Enjoy this nutritious and satisfying chia seed pudding with almond milk as a healthy breakfast, snack, or dessert that aligns with the DASH diet principles and supports renal health.

115. Low•Sodium Veggie Frittata

Ingredient:

- 6 large eggs
- 1/4 cup unsweetened almond milk
- 1/4 tsp black pepper
- 1/8 tsp salt (optional)
- 1 tbsp olive oil
- 1 cup diced bell peppers
- 1 cup diced zucchini
- 1/2 cup diced onion
- 1 cup baby spinach leaves
- 2 tbsp crumbled feta cheese (optional)

Instructions:

1. Preheat the oven to 375°F.

2. In a medium bowl, whisk together the eggs, almond milk, black pepper, and a small amount of salt (if using).

3. In a 9•inch oven•safe non•stick skillet, heat the olive oil over medium heat. Add the diced bell peppers, zucchini, and onion. Sauté for 5•7 minutes, until the vegetables are tender.

4. Add the baby spinach leaves to the skillet and cook for 1•2 minutes, until the spinach is wilted.

5. Pour the egg mixture over the vegetables in the skillet. Gently stir to combine.

6. Transfer the skillet to the preheated oven and bake for 18•22 minutes, or until the frittata is set and lightly golden on top.

7. Remove the frittata from the oven and let it cool for 5 minutes. Slice and serve warm, topped with the crumbled feta cheese (if using).

This low•sodium veggie frittata is a great option for the DASH diet and those following a renal diet. It's high in protein, fiber, and vegetables, while keeping the sodium content low.

The use of unsweetened almond milk and minimal added salt helps to reduce the overall sodium in the dish. The optional feta cheese can be omitted or reduced to further lower the sodium if needed.

Thank you for joining us on this journey to better health with the ***"DASH Diet Cookbook for Renal Health: Maintaining Renal Health with Easy and Delicious DASH Diet Meals."*** We hope this collection of recipes and insights has inspired you to embrace the DASH diet as a valuable tool for supporting your kidney health and overall well-being.

Celebrating Your Commitment to Health

Making the decision to prioritize renal health through diet is a significant and commendable step. By choosing to incorporate the DASH diet into your daily life, you are not only nourishing your body but also taking control of your health in a proactive and meaningful way. The delicious and nutritious recipes in this book are designed to make this journey enjoyable and sustainable, proving that healthy eating can be both flavorful and satisfying.

Reflecting on Your Progress

As you reflect on the recipes you've tried and the meals you've enjoyed, take a moment to appreciate the positive changes you've made. Whether it's improved energy levels, better management of renal conditions, or simply the joy of discovering new favorite dishes, these benefits are a testament to your dedication and effort. Remember, every small step towards healthier eating contributes to a larger goal of maintaining and enhancing your kidney function.

Continuing Your Culinary Adventure

The end of this cookbook is just the beginning of your culinary adventure. Use the recipes and techniques you've learned as a foundation to explore new ingredients, experiment with flavors, and customize meals to suit your preferences and dietary needs. The DASH diet offers a flexible framework that encourages creativity and variety, ensuring that your meals remain exciting and enjoyable.

Staying Informed and Connected

Nutrition science is constantly evolving, and staying informed about the latest research and recommendations can further enhance your journey to renal health. Seek out reputable sources of information, consult with healthcare professionals, and connect with communities that share your commitment to healthy living. By staying engaged and informed, you can continue to make the best choices for your health.

Thank you for allowing us to be a part of your health journey. Here's to a future filled with vitality, well-being, and delicious, kidney-friendly meals!